Carson's
Silent Spring

BLOOMSBURY READER'S GUIDES

Bloomsbury Reader's Guides are clear, concise, and accessible introductions to key texts. Each book explores the themes, context, criticism, and influence of key works, providing a practical introduction to close reading, guiding students towards a thorough understanding of the text. They provide an essential, up-to-date resource, ideal for undergraduate students.

READER'S GUIDES

Carson's *Silent Spring*
A Reader's Guide

JONI SEAGER

BLOOMSBURY
LONDON • NEW DELHI • NEW YORK • SYDNEY

Bloomsbury Academic
An imprint of Bloomsbury Publishing Plc

50 Bedford Square	1385 Broadway
London	New York
WC1B 3DP	NY 10018
UK	USA

www.bloomsbury.com

Bloomsbury is a registered trade mark of Bloomsbury Publishing Plc

First published 2014

© Joni Seager, 2014

Joni Seager has asserted her right under the Copyright, Designs and Patents Act, 1988, to be identified as Author of this work.

All rights reserved. No part of this publication may be reproduced or transmitted in any form or by any means, electronic or mechanical, including photocopying, recording, or any information storage or retrieval system, without prior permission in writing from the publishers.

No responsibility for loss caused to any individual or organization acting on or refraining from action as a result of the material in this publication can be accepted by Bloomsbury or the author.

British Library Cataloguing-in-Publication Data
A catalogue record for this book is available from the British Library.

ISBN: HB: 978-1-4411-1786-1
PB: 978-1-4411-3066-2
ePDF: 978-1-4411-3282-6
ePub: 978-1-4411-2899-7

Library of Congress Cataloging-in-Publication Data
Seager, Joni.
Carson's Silent spring: a reader's guide.
pages cm. — (Reader's guides)
Includes bibliographical references and index.
ISBN 978-1-4411-3066-2 (pbk.) — ISBN 978-1-4411-1786-1 (hardback)
1. Carson, Rachel, 1907-1964. Silent spring. 2. Pesticides—Environmental aspects. 3. Pesticides—Toxicology. 4. Pesticides and wildlife. 5. Insect pests—Biological control. I. Title. II. Title: Silent spring.
QH545.P4C385 2014
363.17'92—dc23
2014002112

Typeset by RefineCatch Limited, Bungay, Suffolk
Printed and bound in Great Britain

Long before it was hip to rage against the machine, Rachel was raging.

Contents

Acknowledgements ix
Note on Source xi

Introducing *Silent Spring*: Hitchcock, Bees, and the Syrian Civil War 1

1 Getting to *Silent Spring* 9

    The making of a publishing bombshell 9
    Author, Author 11

2 The Post-War Machine in the Garden 23

    Control of nature 25
    Science 26
    Science—industry—government collusion 31
    Militaries, militarism, and the atomic world 40
    Crises of confidence 58

3 Needless Havoc: Carson's Case Against Pesticides 67

    The elixirs of death 72
    Thinking like an ecosystem 83
    "Chemical death raining down": Aerial spraying 89
    Cry for the birds 92
    The aquatic holocaust 96
    Pesticides today 98

4 One in Every Four 109
    Domesticating the poisons 111
    Life just not quite fatal 117
    Poison on the plate 119
    The ecology of the body 126
    Disease outcomes 133

5 Alternatives 143
    Passion, wonder, and beauty 143
    Pragmatic alternatives 146
    Scientific uncertainty 152

6 Responses to *Silent Spring* 159
    A book like no other 159
    Stigmatizing perfectly good chemicals* (*and killing Africans at the same time) 166

    Coda 171

Notes 173
Sources for Further Reading and Research 181
Bibliography 183
Index 193

Acknowledgements

The writing of every book "takes a village." I owe many people thanks for supporting, encouraging, and correcting me as I pushed through the seven stages of writing grief—from exhilaration through misgiving and despair (and back again). I would like to acknowledge the many people without whom this book would not have been possible. However, importantly, before I do so, I must say that any remaining errors are my own entirely.

Cynthia Enloe, my partner, is at the heart of all that I do, and without her quick wit, sharp intellect, and unstinting encouragement and support, this, as with so much else, would not have been possible. My friends who were "early readers," Laura Zimmerman, Gilda Bruckman, Candida Lacey, and Madeline Drexler, provided thoughtful feedback on my writing and thinking. And even though I perhaps didn't follow all of their advice at the time, I'm sure they were right—see note about errors, above. My deepest thanks to Julie Clayton who provided expert editorial services that rendered the manuscript into publishable form.

Linda Lear, the eminent biographer of Rachel Carson, gave me warm and unstinting advice, including some cautionary notes on biographical points where I was veering off course, and I have relied heavily on her generosity as well as on her rightly celebrated book, *Rachel Carson: Witness for Nature*. Conservationist Conor Jameson, author of *Silent Spring Revisited*, was generous enough to provide a review of the final draft manuscript; and my thanks also to an anonymous reviewer of the proposal manuscript. William O'Brien at Florida Atlantic University answered astonishingly quickly a few specific queries I posed to him.

Michael Greenwood at Continuum Publishing first suggested that I write a book on *Silent Spring* as part of their *Reader's Guide* series. Continuum later merged with Bloomsbury, and I was soon happily working with Bloomsbury editors Frances Arnold, Rhodri Mogford, and, most importantly, Emily Drewe. Emily provided editorial guidance above and beyond the usual, and I am particularly thankful for her efforts.

I received financial support from my academic institution, Bentley University, for some of the travel and other costs associated with this book, which facilitated its timely completion. I was grateful for opportunities to lecture on *Silent Spring* at the University of Iceland, the U.S. Friends' Higher Education Association, and at the Nordic Geographers' Meeting—venues where I tested and revised some of my ideas.

And, of course, I am most grateful to Rachel Carson herself. An extraordinary woman who persevered and triumphed against many odds, and left a legacy that is unmatched in the annals of environmentalism.

Note on Source

All *Silent Spring* page references are to the 1967 edition, 5th Fawcett Press printing of Rachel Carson's *Silent Spring*. New York: Fawcett Crest. (Original work published 1962 by Houghton Mifflin.)

Silent Spring by Rachel Carson
Copyright © 1962 by Rachel L. Carson
Reprinted by permission of Frances Collin, Trustee

Introducing *Silent Spring*: Hitchcock, Bees, and the Syrian Civil War

In Icelandic, "the voices of spring are silenced": *Raddir vorsins pagna*. In Indonesian, a more poetic double entendre: *Musim Bunga yang Bisu*, "silent spring flowers." In English, *Silent Spring*. Not **The** *Silent Spring*, which might suggest a singular and perhaps passing event, a one-time seasonal aberration. Rather, a simple, bold, unflinching, unmediated warning of a mute death about to settle upon us.

For most of us, unexpected silence is profoundly unsettling. Silence is impenetrable, incomprehensible. The tensest scenes in horror movies are not those filled with screams and moans or even eerie music; the most unbearable anticipation of terror creeps in under cover of deep silence. Alfred Hitchcock, Carson's contemporary, knew this; he made silence into high horror cinema art. Carson was no psychoanalyst, and there's no evidence that she knew Hitchcock, or even liked his films, but she brilliantly tapped, as did he, a deep vein of human dread by invoking silence.

In a two-word title, *Silent Spring*, Carson signaled the dark warning of her book: that "man-made" chemicals were killing the harbingers of spring, of life itself. Birds, but not only birds—insects, fish, domestic animals: all dead or dying; all mute. In the season when we teeter on the edge of our winter-weary seats, straining for the first raucousness of rebirth and reawakening, no raucousness, no noise; instead, a slowly rising panic of silence. And then Carson drops the other shoe: "No witchcraft, no enemy action had silenced the rebirth of new life in this stricken world. The people had done it themselves" (p. 14). As the comic-strip character Pogo would say a decade later on Earth Day 1971, surveying a scene of environmental devastation, "we have met the enemy and he is us."

Rachel Carson was heralded and hated in the wake of *Silent Spring*. Following its 1962 US release, *Silent Spring* raced around the world in more than 20 foreign-language translations, from Arabic to Swedish, and publication in dozens of countries. Worldwide book sales quickly reached the hundreds of thousands, and now, still mounting, are counted literally in the millions. Serialized, reviewed, and excerpted in uncountable numbers of journals, magazines, TV, and radio shows, *Silent Spring* reached even further into popular culture and consciousness.

Carson herself became a pivotal figure—symbolically, and as an actual agent of change—in the wrenching cultural clashes of the 1960s. Succumbing to health impacts related to breast cancer in 1964, she lived long enough after *Silent Spring*'s publication to receive the full brunt of attack, but not to witness the full force of its transformative effect. And what a transformation! *Silent Spring*—not by itself, but signally—launched a new consciousness, a new regulatory approach to synthetic chemicals, and a new way of conceptualizing humans' place in the ecological web. But I'm getting ahead of myself.

Silent Spring is often talked about these days in rather hushed tones as a "classic." What that usually means is that most people think they should have read it—perhaps even believe they have read it, at some moment in the hazy past—but in fact have not. A "classic" tends to sit petulantly on the shelf; there because its dimly-remembered merits earned its claim to shelf space, or perhaps there because the owner wishes to *be seen* making the claim of owning it. But a classic tends to sit mostly unperturbed.

In an amusing anecdote, Sandra Steingraber, a noted biologist and environmentalist, confesses this common experience. On being asked in 1990 to give a lecture on Carson for Earth Day, she recalls:

> I reread *Silent Spring*. Or at least I initially thought I was rereading it. The words in the yellowing copy that I had on my bookshelf—

probably bequeathed to me by my father—didn't sound familiar to me at all. I could not, upon further reflection, recall ever having been assigned to read the book by any professor in any of the many ecology and environmental classes I had ever taken. So, by chapter four, I was forced to conclude, with head-hanging shame, that I had never before actually read the damn book and that any flashes of recognition I felt were because Carson was forever being quoted by other authors in other books.

(Steingraber, 2008, p. 222)

***

In Carson's case, shelf-bound classic status notwithstanding, the importance of the work, remarkably and resiliently, continues to roll forward: more than 50 years after its publication, *Silent Spring* continues to be invoked in contemporary debates about climate change, mosquito control, public health, and ethics. Carson's warnings about the ecological catastrophe being wrought by the wanton use and misuse of pesticides seem more salient today than ever. In spring 2010, the United States' "President's Cancer Panel" released its annual report for 2008–2009—the first one to focus on the links between environment and cancer. The 240-page report doesn't mention Rachel Carson by name, but her work informs every page. The report asserts that environmental cancers are "grossly underestimated" and "needlessly devastate American lives"; that the regulatory approach is reactive not precautionary; that harmful effects of exposure to synthetic chemicals occur at low doses; and that a lack of regulatory will, combined with "undue industry influence," renders ineffective regulation of environmental contaminants. It's an alarming commentary that 50-plus years after *Silent Spring*, this can be cast as news. What the President's Cancer Panel doesn't address is the carnage to animals, birds, and ecosystems from pesticides, that makes *Silent Spring* so heartbreaking to read. Carson pleads against the "vogue for poisons" and the "habit of killing . . . any creature that may annoy or inconvenience us" (p. 117).

As I write this in summer 2013, two pesticide-related catastrophes have captured global news headlines, and in both stories *Silent Spring* resonates loudly:

In June 2013, shoppers in Wilsonville, Oregon, discovered piles of dead and dying bees, eventually tallying more than 50,000, in a local parking lot. Coming in the midst of mounting global anxiety about the fate of pollinators (and of the agriculture that depends on them), this, the world's largest recorded single die-off of bumblebees, was shocking enough to catch national and international attention. What particularly piqued interest and alarm is the fact that the bees were killed in such an ordinary way, by an everyday occurrence: it turns out that a landscaping company sprayed linden trees in the parking lot with a popular insecticide—brand name "Safari" (active killing ingredient, "dinotefuran")—trying to kill aphids on the trees. The trees were flowering, bees came to collect the pollen, and contact with the pesticide produced certain death among them—for many of them protracted and painful.

Safari (dinotefuran) belongs to a class of insecticides called "neonicotinoids." Chemically related to nicotine, a plant with natural insecticidal qualities, neonicotinoids are one of the few new classes of insecticides developed in the past 50 years. The neonicotinoids were developed (originally by Shell Oil in the 1980s, and then Bayer in the 1990s) in some measure because they were proven to be less toxic to mammals, including humans, compared with "old" insecticides such as organophosphates. But they are more toxic to bees (and many other insects). Such bee toxicity is alarming in its own right, but also has drawn wide attention since bees are absolutely central to food production, and unimaginable declines in bee populations in the past decade are threatening global food supplies. Neonicotinoids have been temporarily banned in several jurisdictions, including the European Union, but the manufacturers of neonicotinoids are fighting a fierce battle against bans.

Valent USA (a subsidiary of Sumitomo Chemicals, Japan), the manufacturer of Safari, advertises it on its website as "a super-systemic insecticide with quick uptake and knockdown," under a banner advertising headline proclaiming "Safari Insecticide. *Where the wild things aren't*" (emphasis in original).[1] The company apparently isn't perturbed by the irony of such claims in the aftermath of their pesticide being responsible for the world's largest single-event bee killing.

A local ecologist organized a memorial service for the bees in Oregon, saying: "This isn't a funeral. We're not there to bury the bees or build little bee coffins. We're going there to talk about what this means."[2] Carson would have a lot to add to that conversation, and I'm sure *Silent Spring* was invoked many times during the community gathering. Carson—even writing, as she was, in what we now think of as the early days of the pesticide revolution—was acutely aware of the mounting chemical threats to bees, and throughout *Silent Spring* warns against their destruction (including a particularly poignant description in Chapter 10 of the destruction of several colonies of bees through DDT aerial spraying). Many of the news reports about the Oregon 2013 bee kill invoked *Silent Spring*, some asking rhetorically "and just how long has it been since Carson wrote that book?"

In July 2013, 23 schoolchildren in Dharmasati Gandaman, a village in Bihar state, India, were killed and dozens more hospitalized after being poisoned by their school-provided hot lunch that was contaminated by a pesticide. The exact means of contamination remains, as I write, unclear. The first news reports suggested that the lunch was prepared with oil that was stored in a container that previously had been used to store the pesticide. But a week after the deaths, investigators suggested the more shocking possibility that a bottle of the pesticide may have been inadvertently used in the food preparation instead of a bottle of cooking oil.[3] The lethal ingredient stirred into the food was monocrotophos, a highly toxic organophosphate insecticide. Monocrotophos has been banned in dozens of countries, including Australia, Cambodia, China, the European Union, Indonesia, Laos, Philippines, Sri Lanka, Thailand, Vietnam, and the United States, but remains widely available in India.

Organophosphates are, by now, "old" pesticides, developed in the 1930s. They work by disrupting the central nervous system, and in World War II the German military discovered that organophosphates made highly effective chemical weapons. Many militaries today still store—and some deploy—chemical weapons such as sarin that use concentrated amounts of organophosphate compounds. For example, evidence strongly supports accusations that the ruling Assad government in Syria used chemical weapons against their opponents in the civil war raging there. The Assad regime's chemical weapon of choice appears to be sarin (an organophosphate), also a favorite weapon used by Saddam Hussein in Iraq. The history and the chemical composition of chemical weapons and of pesticides are inextricably woven together—a point that Carson makes in *Silent Spring*. Many pesticides and military chemical weapons were developed from the same research and developmental process, sometimes literally in the same laboratory, and their uses, if not always simultaneously developed, were often developed hand-in-glove.

In rural India, organophosphate pesticides are ubiquitous—thus the likelihood is strong that in an agricultural state such as Bihar, a container formerly used to store pesticides or, indeed, a bottle of the pesticide itself, would be readily at hand and could make its way into the food-preparation chain. Vandana Shiva, India's most prominent environmentalist, describes her country as "drowning in pesticides."[4] Indeed, organophosphate-based pesticides are *so* common in rural areas in India, and elsewhere, that they are commonly used in suicides. A 2008 study in the British medical journal, *Lancet*, established that more than 200,000 people a year worldwide commit suicide with organophosphates alone—and many more are injured trying to do so (Eddleston et al., 2008). Another study a few years earlier pegged the total number of global suicide pesticide deaths at about 300,000 (Gunnell and Eddleston, 2003). In India, suicide-by-pesticide has recently become common among male farmers, although suicide rates in rural areas of India are highest among young women under age 24 (Gunnell and Eddleston, 2003). In China—the only country with a higher overall rate of female suicide than male (mostly young, rural women)—62 percent of suicide deaths were the result of ingesting pesticides or rat poison. The authors of a recent epidemiological study make the point that "[y]oung women in most countries tend to have high rates of attempting suicide, but easy access to pesticide and rat poison in rural areas of China may account for the high fatality rate" (Yip and Liu, 2006). In a few horrifying cases documented in India and Afghanistan (and widely suspected elsewhere), women have been murdered by being forced to drink pesticides in a form of chemical "honor killing." Of course, unknown more thousands are killed each year in unintentional poisonings wherever organophosphate (and other) pesticides are readily available. The 23 children in Bihar just happened to have caught the attention of the global media.

In Chapter 3 of *Silent Spring*, "Elixirs of Death," Carson previews much of this. Interestingly, in light of the contemporary global epidemic of suicide-by-pesticide, she mentions the "popularity" of organic phosphates (at that time, parathion especially) among people committing suicide in Finland; in the same section, she highlights the lethality of parathion to bees.[5] But her overarching primary message in this section of *Silent Spring* is about the dangers of accidental and unwitting contact (often through misuse or reuse of containers) with organic phosphate pesticides, and she enumerates the tally of accidental deaths attributed to just one, parathion— including in India; even when she was writing, pesticide deaths in India were striking. As we will see, Carson was also ahead of her time in focusing attention on the militarized links in today's pesticide chain. She was one of the first to draw attention to the militarized origins of pesticides, and throughout *Silent Spring* she offers a trenchant critique of the militarization not only of pesticides, but of human relations to nature.

***

As much as it seems that *Silent Spring* is vindicated by contemporary events, it remains a highly controversial book. Indeed, in the early years of the twenty-first century, there is a resurgence of personal animus directed at Rachel Carson herself; she is being publicly excoriated in forums ranging from India's law courts to the US Congress and the United Nations. As I explore in Chapter 6, the right-wing conservative movement in the United States has launched a concerted effort to rehabilitate DDT and to damn Carson all over again. The battles Carson fought are raging still—or, again. Carson might be bemused to see *Silent Spring* bestowed "honorable mention" status on a 2005 US political conservative listing of the "Ten Most Harmful Books of the 19th and 20th Centuries"(Human Events, 2005)—keeping company with *The Feminine Mystique*, *Communist Manifesto*, and *Mein Kampf*.

Silent Spring has become a Rorschach test. Across the span of time since its publication in 1962, the meaning of *Silent Spring* has been stretched impossibly beyond its original shape. Like the old-fashioned party game, "telephone," in which a message whispered from one ear to another reaches the tenth person so garbled (often hilariously so) that it is no longer comprehensible, *Silent Spring* has become a canvas onto which we impose all kinds of arguments and meanings, and *assumed* meanings, some of which have strayed very far from the original intent.

On the one hand, this points to the brilliance of Carson and her book—that they remain so pliably relevant for so long. But it also means that the core insights, the core arguments, and the originality of *Silent Spring* are being left behind. Walking back to a core document can be a sobering and exhilarating journey. This book is intended to be a guide along that journey.

1

Getting to *Silent Spring*

The making of a publishing bombshell

Silent Spring appeared in print for the first time as a three-part serialization in *The New Yorker* magazine in June 1962. This was a brilliant publishing strategy—both for Carson and for *The New Yorker*. For Carson, the serialization built interest in the book that was released three months later, and it put her ideas directly into the living rooms of a broad audience but especially of the national elite. Carson had forged this publishing strategy with earlier books, and by the late 1950s she had become a nationally recognized and admired writer in large part because she wrote for popular outlets. While Carson was always attentive to sustaining her credentials as a professional scientist, she published liberally for what we would call today "crossover" and popular audiences. Throughout the 1950s, she wrote regularly for outlets such as *Nature, Collier's,* and *Reader's Digest,* among others, and in serialization for *The New Yorker*.

For *The New Yorker*, publishing *Silent Spring* helped secure the reputation it was then building as a go-to source for investigative reporting and as the preeminent national "big ideas" forum. In 1946, they had broken new reportorial territory by devoting an entire issue to John Hersey's *Hiroshima*, a searing account of the effects of the US nuclear bomb dropped on Japan. Following *Silent Spring*, in 1963 they brought Hannah Arendt's five-part reportage of the trial of Nazi Adolf Eichmann to a shocked American audience. A decade after running the *Silent Spring* essays, *The New Yorker* catapulted itself again into the front of the national discussion by running several full-length investigatory reports by Seymour Hersh exposing the US massacre of Vietnamese civilians—and other atrocities—at My Lai, Ky Chanh, and Son My.

But running *Silent Spring* in 1962 took particular fortitude. *The New Yorker* and Carson had built their previous successful relationship on the basis of two of her earlier works that they had serialized, *The Edge of the Sea* (1955) and *The Sea Around Us* (1951). These were primarily descriptive naturalist writings: lyrical, beautiful, scientifically based, but "safe" writings of the "wonders of nature" genre; these books did not enter any polemic or make any argument as such. (Although both books did draw attention to the threats to the marine environment by human activities, they did so in a more subliminal and subtle way).

Silent Spring, by comparison, was a call to arms, a hard-hitting exposé of human calumny, a big-picture, naming-names investigation of devastating implications. Prior to its June release in *The New Yorker*, Carson had circulated chapters of *Silent Spring* to colleagues for peer review, and had started to talk about the book at selected meetings and conferences. This advance activity stirred considerable interest, and also spurred rumors and leaks (many misguided) about what "Miss Carson's" book would be saying about chemicals and pesticides. At least one chemical company, Velsicol, directly threatened *The New Yorker* and Houghton Mifflin (the book publisher) with a lawsuit if it moved forward with publication; and another, DuPont, was making threatening noises in the same direction. Largely due to their confidence in the prior legal and scientific review they had prudently commissioned, and due to the personal commitment of William Shawn (the editor at *The New Yorker*) and Paul Brooks (editor-in-chief at Houghton Mifflin), both publishers held firm against mounting pressure to pull or alter the release.

And the rest, as they say, is history. *Silent Spring* burst onto the American scene in late 1962 with unprecedented effect. Once the book was out, there was no turning away, no going back. The world, in many ways, can be divided into "before *Silent Spring*" and "after."

One of the intriguing questions is "Why?" *Silent Spring* is a fine book, excruciatingly researched, wonderfully written and composed, gripping reading. But it was not the first "important" environmental book of its time. Jacque Cousteau's blockbuster, *The Silent World*

(1953) was an astonishingly successful bestseller (for which Carson, identified as "the author of *The Sea Around Us*," wrote a rather restrained book-jacket endorsement, "it had my fascinated attention . . ."), but Cousteau's success did not launch a revolution.[1] Eugene Odum's 1953 *Fundamentals of Ecology*, despite its leaden title, *was* revolutionary—in pioneering the notion of "ecosystem" and laying out the elements of holistic ecosystems understanding—but its influence remained largely confined to academia. Murray Bookchin, writing under the name of Lewis Herber, published *Our Synthetic Environment* in 1962, a wider-ranging exploration of chemicals in the environment than *Silent Spring*, but it garnered very little public attention. Throughout the 1950s, physicist Gilbert Plass made urgent predictions in popular magazines such as *Time* (1953), as well as scientific outlets such as *American Scientist* (1956), about global warming caused by industrial pollution, but his work gained little traction. Yet *Silent Spring* took the world by storm.

Author, Author

Carson herself, of course, is the central character in the story of the making of this publishing bestseller. A brief snapshot of Carson's adult life reveals how complicated and challenging it was. She was a woman who was the sole breadwinner for a complicated household that, over many years, consisted of several dependent relatives, including a young nephew for whom she was an adoptive parent; who juggled family and economic demands while writing four books (as well as dozens of articles and essays); who was a skilled field biologist; who remained single her entire life but was engaged in a decade-long love affair (of some uncertain nature) with a married woman; who took on the most entrenched and powerful interests and institutions—all while battling uphill against the gender discrimination of her era and the ferocious misogyny that followed the publication of *Silent Spring,* and who did so while dealing with a series of escalating health problems ending with a several-year struggle with breast cancer.

The facts of Carson's life are now well known, and I won't spend much time covering terrain that is already well mapped (see, especially, Lear, 2009). Carson was born in rural Pennsylvania in 1907, the youngest of three children. Her mother, who became her adult companion and one of her most devoted friends, inculcated in her daughter a curiosity and love for nature, encouraging Carson to explore the natural world around her. Despite the constant financial precariousness of her family, Carson was able to attend college; she graduated from Pennsylvania College for Women (now Chatham College) in 1929, studied at Woods Hole Marine Biological Laboratory, and received her MA in Zoology from Johns Hopkins University in 1932. It is of passing interest to note that Gertrude Stein, another Pennsylvanian-born woman bound for fame and notoriety, also studied at Woods Hole and then Johns Hopkins, some 30 years before Carson. The reason that Stein, Carson, and literally hundreds of other women, many of whom became prominent scientists, cycled through the Marine Biological Laboratory at Woods Hole was because it was one of the few scientific institutions that welcomed women in the early years of the twentieth century and treated them as equal participants in science. Both Woods Hole and Carson benefited from their brief association. In 2013, Woods Hole erected a statue commemorating Carson, a life-sized bronze model of her sitting on the dock, notebook in hand, looking out at the sea.

Carson was a skilled writer—she entered college as an English major before her mentor, Mary Scott Skinker, lured her away into the study of biology. With this unusual combination of skill in both science and writing, she was hired by the US Bureau of Fisheries[2] to write radio scripts during the Depression, and she supplemented her income by writing feature articles on natural history for the *Baltimore Sun* newspaper. In 1936, she began a 16-year career as a scientist and editor for the US Fish and Wildlife Service, eventually rising to the position of editor-in-chief of all the agency's publications.

For the Fish and Wildlife Service she wrote pamphlets on conservation and natural resources, synthesized field reports on fisheries into brochures, and edited scientific articles. She also continued her freelancing life: her first national-audience commercial success was an article, "Undersea" (1937), which she wrote for the *Atlantic Monthly*. This was received to such acclaim that it was the basis of *Under the Sea-Wind* (1941), a book that garnered good reviews but never sold particularly well. In 1951, she published her lyrical study of the ocean, *The Sea Around Us*. This book leapt to *The New York Times* bestseller list, where it remained for almost 90 weeks, it won the National Book Award, it was condensed in *Reader's Digest*, and it made Carson a household name. *The Sea Around Us* also gave her the financial independence she needed to resign from government service in 1952 to devote herself full time to her writing. In 1955, she followed the success of *The Sea Around Us* with a study of the coastal Atlantic, *The Edge of the Sea*—retrospectively, the third of a three-part "biography of the ocean." By the time *The Edge of the Sea* was released, Carson was famous.

A 1951 review of *The Sea Around Us* starts off with a casual observation that "Rachel Carson is a marine biologist who wears the unlikely title of editor-in-chief of the United States Fish and Wildlife Service" (Leonard, 1951). "Unlikely"? That a woman would be an editor-in-chief? That a woman would be a professional at the Fish and Wildlife Service? While the reviewer seems to insert this comment somewhat snidely, his observation could be read merely as a stark acknowledgement of workforce realities. In 1950 in the United States, only 34 percent of women worked in the paid workforce (compared with 86 percent of men); of the total civilian labor force in 1950, 70 percent of workers were men (Toossi, 2002). Few women working for wages in the 1940s were "professionals"; the majority held clerical or service jobs. This gender skew was even more prominent in the sciences. In the 1940s, when Carson was actively employed as a scientist, only about 4 percent of the scientists listed in the American government's "National Roster of Scientific and Specialized Personnel" were women (Rossiter, 1998, p. 25).

Carson's choice of the sciences, then, was an unusual one for a woman in the 1930s (indeed, to a large extent, it is still so today). By the middle of World War II, a decade after Carson started out on her quest as a working scientist, with looming *man*power shortages, women were being pressed into service in any number of new occupations, even in the sciences (see Rossiter, 1998). Throughout the war, women made significant contributions in a number of science fields, including the most highly masculinized fields such as physics and engineering; but this was still viewed widely as an anomaly— and after the war, women were supposed to relinquish their jobs to the men returning from military service. This "Rosie the Riveter" phenomenon cut across all occupations. But as a single woman and sole provider for her family, Carson was not in a position to relinquish her job to anyone, and she remained employed by the Fish and Wildlife Service until 1952, when she was sufficiently established as a writer that she could support herself on her writing income.

Carson remained single her entire life. As an adult woman in mid-twentieth-century America, this put her in a distinct—and stereotyped as odd—minority. Statistically speaking, Carson should have married in 1930—23 being the median age of first marriage for white women at that time (it is now about 27) (Elliot et al., 2012). Rather than marrying in 1930, Carson was just then launching her graduate work at Johns Hopkins in the Zoology department, having graduated from the Pennsylvania College for Women the previous summer. Her family was in a precarious financial state, and Carson was responsible for five "partially dependent" family members (Lear, 2009, p. 76). In 1930, Carson was juggling school loans, part-time teaching assistantships, economic responsibility for her extended family household, and squirrels for her laboratory research who refused to breed. Not only was Rachel *not* marrying, there were no signs of boyfriends or dating or any interest in bringing yet more people into her complicated life. Biographer Linda Lear reports that most of Carson's classmates during this period remembered Rachel as "an unattractive girl who kept entirely to herself, studied all the time, and had few friends" (Lear, 2009, p. 497).

Despite this rather starch view, Carson was not friendless for most of her life. Indeed, throughout her life, she forged long and enduring bonds with loyal friends—many of whom were the women who mentored her and who supported her interest in the sciences when Carson would have found little support elsewhere. Women such as Mary Skinker (her professor), Marie Rodell (her literary agent), Shirley Briggs (a colleague from Fish and Wildlife), Marjorie Spock (a community activist against pesticides), Ida Sprow (her housekeeper), Olga Huckins (the naturalist who brought Carson into the world of pesticides): these were the friends who sustained her throughout her life—a cadre of fiercely loyal and protective friends who never failed her.

And then there was Dorothy Freeman. She met Dorothy and Dorothy's husband, Stan, in 1953, when Carson moved to a house she had newly bought for herself by the sea in Southport, Maine. Rachel and Dorothy found themselves entranced with one another;

there was an instant chemistry between them, and Rachel came quickly to feel that Dorothy was her soul mate. They were launched on what would be a decade-long loving relationship that was by far the most intimate and most central relationship in each of their lives. It was an overtly romantic relationship, a physically close one, and a relationship of two hearts and minds melded. Whether it was also a sexual relationship—truly what we would call a "lesbian" relationship—remains, looking back with our twenty-first-century sensibilities, unknown, unknowable, and contested. Rachel and Dorothy were physically close, often spending snatched nights together at hotels when Rachel was on the road doing talks, squeezing out time in between summers in Maine. When they were not together, they wrote to each other at a frenetic pace. The letters piled up, sometimes several a day. They developed a system of writing, sometimes, two-part letters—the first, a general letter that could be shared with Rachel's mother or Dorothy's husband, the second tucked inside for their private reading (Lear, 2009, p. 252).

Many of their letters survived, but most were destroyed. On at least one occasion, Rachel and Dorothy together burned a packet of letters; others were destroyed singly and separately, though often by mutual agreement (Freeman, 1995, p. xvi). The surviving letters were compiled by Dorothy's granddaughter and published in 1995 (Freeman, 1995). The letters give tremendous insight into Rachel's creative process, the swirl that engulfed her life both before and after *Silent Spring*, and, always, they speak clearly of the love of these two women. Rachel and Dorothy, themselves, seemed not quite sure what to make of their relationship. In one letter, Rachel wrote:

> What I feel most clearly is that we must never again for a moment forget what a precious possession we have in our love and understanding, and in that constant and sometimes almost puzzling longing to share with each other every thought and experience . . . If ever I have seemed to forget the wonder and fragile beauty of it, darling, know that I won't forget again.
>
> (Freeman, 1995, p. xx)

At this distance, and with the walls of privacy drawn high around their relationship, perhaps our best lens for viewing it is as a version of a "Boston marriage." Lillian Faderman, in her remarkable book on the many forms that women's intimate relationships with one another take, *Surpassing The Love of Men*, describes a Boston marriage this way:

> The term "Boston marriage" was used in late nineteenth-century New England to describe a long-term monogamous relationship between two otherwise unmarried women. The women were generally financially independent . . . they were usually feminists, New Women, often pioneers in a profession. They were also very involved in culture and in social betterment, and these female values, which they shared with each other, formed a basis for their life together. Their relationships were in every sense, as described by a Bostonian Mark DeWolfe Howe, the nineteenth-century *Atlantic Monthly* editor . . . a "union – there is no truer word for it." Whether these unions sometimes or often included sex we will never know, but we do know that these women spent their lives primarily with other women, they gave to other women the bulk of their energy and attention, and they formed powerful emotional ties with other women. If their personalities could be projected to our times, it is probable that they would see themselves as "women-identified women," i.e., what we would call lesbians, regardless of the level of their sexual interests.
>
> (Faderman, 1981, p. 190)

To the public, however, Carson was a "spinster." This position as a "spinster" played variously to her advantage and disadvantage throughout her career. On the one hand, an unmarried, middle-class white woman such as Carson could be viewed as a stock figure of reliability and respectability in the middle of the twentieth century. To many outward appearances, Rachel represented a modest, no-nonsense woman who was briskly and efficiently running her own household, complete with her mother who lived with her throughout much of her adult life. Such a woman was easily typecast as "sensible" and stable. The role she forged for herself as a writer of "nature appreciation" essays and books, fits well with this restrained image, and the two images—spinster and nature appreciator—supported one another in solidifying her public identity as a much admired and "safe," even sentimental, science writer. In her obituary, *The New York Times* referred to her reputation as "the essence of gentle scholarship" (Obituary, *The New York Times*, 1964). Contemporaries, apparently not uncommonly, referred to her as the "nun of nature" (Griswold, 2012), a peculiar backhanded compliment. A 1951 review of *The Sea Around Us* referred to her, admiringly, as "the slender, gentle Miss Carson" (cited in Dreier, 2012, p. 229), while another review by the science editor of *Time* magazine reassured readers that Carson's book about sea life was "charming," that the animals she described were her "friends" whom she loved, and that the very ocean currents themselves were "dear to her"; he concluded his genteelly paternalistic review wondering what Carson looked like (there was no photo of her on the book's dust jacket), saying, "It would be pleasant to know what a woman looks like who can write about exacting science with such beauty and precision" (Leonard, 1951). One can almost feel the pat on the head.

On the other hand, as Carson ventured into more contested terrain with her work leading up to *Silent Spring*, and then with the publication itself, and started to challenge powerful interests and institutions, her "spinsterism" was wielded against her. Her critics responded as though being an unmarried, middle-aged woman was a disease or at least a disability. As we'll see in Chapter 6, many of the most ferocious attacks on Carson after *Silent Spring* drew attention to her identity as an unmarried woman—both of which, critics argued, undercut her competence. That a mere woman, let alone a "spinster," should be taken seriously on scientific matters was unimaginable! The critics were drawing on a long tradition of disdain and distrust of women who did not fulfill the cultural expectations of "normal" womanhood; the spinster stereotype as a deviant and slightly unhinged woman was a cheap and easily accessible cultural stereotype for Carson's critics to invoke (Faderman, 1981; Faludi, 1991; Mustard, 2000). One can only imagine the hysterical condemnation that would have ensued if her intimate relationship with Freeman were made public.

This wild pendulum swing in the interpretation of Carson's identity is not unfamiliar to women in science—now, as then.

As long as Carson was sticking with the "lyrically written, evocative, poetic" descriptions of life in the sea and on the edge of the sea, she was in safe womanly territory. As soon as she started to challenge industrial, agricultural, government, and consumer interests—raising, indeed, a challenge to the entire American "way of life"—she was breaking gender bounds and the bounds of social tolerance for women scientists. Sentimentality, subjectivity, feelings: these are all "normal" womanly attributes, and not really the domain of science. Reason and objectivity: these are male domains, and are cherished as the core attributes of science. As contemporary scientist Evelyn Fox Keller makes clear, the association of women with sentimentality and feelings has long been used as a rationale for excluding them from science—normative science has no room for feelings, we are taught (Keller, 1985). Carson was often caught between the two: trying to combine science with feeling, she had to fight against the predominant idea of her time, that science and spirit were separate (Hazlett, 2008). To a large extent, with her first three books, Carson succeeded in bridging these two solitudes, which no doubt contributed to their enthusiastic public reception. But as Carson swung away from her early "nature writing" into a reasoned polemic against vested interests, she was moving out of "normal" womanly range and into contested male territory. And the response—both positive and negative—was fierce.

The genteel art of careful nature observation has a long history as a socially acceptable avocation—and, at times, vocation—for women. Historians of science have identified botany, especially, as one of the few socially acceptable scientific fields, over several centuries, acceptable for women. As Ann Shteir establishes, "As early as the 1700's women had more culturally sanctioned access to botany than to any other science: they collected plants, drew them, studied them, and named them, taught their children about plants, and wrote popularizing books on botany. Botany came to be widely associated with women and was widely gender coded as feminine" (Shteir, 1997). Observing and writing about the "charms" of nature—most accessible in descriptions of plants, especially flowers—were considered suitable undertakings for women even in pre-Victorian times (see also Jackson-Houlston, 2006).

Although women were excluded from botany as it professionalized and was consciously reshaped as a male field in the late 1800s, the genteel association of women and "nature appreciation," broadly understood, remained. Sandra Harding's work on standpoint theory underscores the ways in which the social organization of science is gendered, and makes the point that norms about appropriate scientific interests for women and men are culturally and temporally specific (see, for example, Harding, 1997). In these terms, botany and nature appreciation represented a harmony of what Shteir calls "gender and genre." Strains of this unthreatening association are evident in the reviews of Carson's early books on the sea. For many readers and reviewers of Carson's pre-*Silent Spring* books (such as the *Time* science editor quoted above), a spinster writing nature essays was the very epitome of "safe" and "reassuring" in a quite Victorian way.

Carson herself would have eschewed this association, perhaps even been horrified by it. She viewed herself as a working scientist, a field biologist, and a trained naturalist; no mere "flower appreciator," she. And yet in many ways she remained confined by the gender conventions of the mid-twentieth century, and to the extent that she broke barriers, she did so relatively imperceptibly—or, at least, imperceptibly to her general readership—until *Silent Spring*. Carson was well aware of the precarious position she occupied as a woman scientist, and was ambivalent, herself, about how to reconcile the two. In a 1951 speech to *The New York Herald Tribune* Book and Author Luncheon, she may have surprised her audience by these remarks:

> People often seem to be surprised that a woman has written a book about the sea. This is especially true, I find, of men. Perhaps they have been accustomed to thinking of the more exciting fields of scientific knowledge as exclusively masculine domains. Then even if they accept my sex, some people are further surprised to find that I am not a tall, oversize, Amazon-type female. I can offer no defense for not being what people expect, but perhaps I might say a few words about why a woman, and only an average-size one at that, should have become a biographer of the sea.
>
> (cited in Lear, 2009, p. 214)

What was not fully appreciated at the time—indeed perhaps not until the 1980s—was the extent to which Carson broke ground in the *environmental* field. As Patricia Hynes notes:

> Until *Silent Spring*, women were the second sex in the conservation and environmental movement . . . Carson severed the tradition of only men having the big ideas and setting the agenda in the environmental movement. Not being the wife or the colleague of some great man, she was preserved from absorption into a man's career. Her work cannot be collapsed into someone else's.
>
> (Hynes, 1989, p. 50)

Carson was a fierce advocate for her own interests and was particularly canny about publishing. In 1948, as Carson was writing her second book, *The Sea Around Us*, she was introduced to Marie Rodell, a literary agent with whom she struck up a lifelong friendship and business partnership. She and Rodell were a formidable team. Together they crafted brilliant publishing strategies (and contracts) that were instrumental in shaping Carson's publishing career. But even with Rodell on board, Carson remained alert to her own publishing interests and promotion—a role that she took to energetically, pressing for direct involvement in the production and promotion of her books. For example, Carson continuously sent Oxford University Press suggestions for the promotion of her book with them, *The Sea Around Us*. She paid attention to the binding, to the quality of printing, to the cover art; nothing was too small to escape her notice. In a letter in March 1951 to Catherine Scott, Oxford's head of public relations, she complained, "[The paper binding] cheapens an otherwise handsomely made book, and is hardly appropriate for anything but a book you are going to read once then throw away" (Messier, 2012); she continued in similar vein over several weeks, keeping an eagle eye on Oxford's handling of her book. As Linda Lear notes:

> Rachel's involvement in the physical production of *The Sea Around Us* was more than mere professional interest. Her efforts to influence the marketing in particular were symptomatic of the perfectionism that she demanded of herself as well as of the control she wanted over all aspects of her writing.
>
> (Lear, 2009, p. 192)

Rodell and Carson were equally sophisticated about crafting and protecting Carson's public image as a knowledgeable scientist, and cultivating her reputation as a public intellectual "reliable narrator" about the natural world. Between them, they forged a formidable platform from which Carson changed the world.

2

The Post-War Machine in the Garden

In 1956, as Carson was starting to engage directly with the research that would yield *Silent Spring*, an American Studies scholar, Leo Marx, published an article called "The Machine in the Garden" (Marx, 1956). In 1964, he extended his analysis in a book by the same evocative title, a book that became a surprising hit. *The Machine in the Garden* has remained in print ever since. Marx and Carson, though contemporaries, were unlikely to have ever met, and their fields and interests seem quite far apart, but in many ways their work mirrored one another's and reflected an emerging temper of the times. Leo Marx's analysis was a literary and historical one, tracing through literature the eighteenth- and nineteenth-century intrusion into and transformation of American pastoralism and pastoral ideals by industrialization. The literal machines of early industrial capitalism—including factories, railways, and mechanical agricultural machines—were overtaking earlier sensibilities and ways of life, altering social and economic relations, and transforming conventions of human encounters with their environment. "The machine" was as much a habit of mind as a mechanic. As capitalist industrialization overtook the agrarian and pastoral American pre-industrial society, Marx argues, one unmistakable outcome was a growing detachment and "unrelatedness" to nature—as well as to a sense of social cohesion and a common good.

Leo Marx was explicitly examining the ways that "the machine" transformed, irrevocably, American life and culture. At first glance, Carson was not. *Silent Spring,* supposedly, is mostly about pesticides.

But Carson's book was much more than a polemic against pesticides. At its heart, *Silent Spring* is a manifesto against "the machine in the garden."

In an Afterword he wrote for a later edition of his book (1999), Leo Marx makes the link between his analysis and Carson's, particularly drawing attention to the way Carson frames her opening scene as a peaceful pastoral idyll about to be shattered by an external force—metaphorically, by the machine. Carson's opening sentence of her opening chapter, "A Fable for Tomorrow," sets the stage of a quintessentially American pastoral scene: "There once was a town in the heart of America where all life seemed to live in harmony with its surroundings" (p. 13). She paints an idyllic picture of foxes frolicking, deer leaping through misty fields, ferns and wildflowers flourishing; people in happy harmony with the land. This is an abundant and life-giving landscape, Carson continues, essentially unchanged since the first settlers. But then, abruptly, the tone shifts as the "machine" approaches:

> [A] strange blight crept over the area . . . Some evil spell had settled on the community: mysterious maladies swept the flocks of chickens; the cattle and sheep sickened and died. Everywhere was a shadow of death . . . The few birds seen anywhere were moribund: they trembled violently and could not fly. On the mornings that had once throbbed with the dawn chorus of robins, catbirds, doves, jays, wrens, and scores of other bird voices there was no new sound; only silence lay over the fields and woods and marsh.
>
> (pp. 13–14)

Carson goes on to paint a fuller picture of the sudden devastation. There were no blooms on the apple trees, no fish in the rivers, no chickens hatched, litters of pigs died. A clue to the mystery, Carson suggests, is a peculiar "white granular powder" (p. 14) that had appeared a few weeks prior and had settled into the eaves and gutters on the rooftops; a powder of death. This is "the machine."

Before it was hip to rage against the machine, Carson was raging.

Control of nature

Carson's meta-narrative was not about pesticides, but about the control of nature; or, rather, about the havoc and destruction that humans unleash in their efforts—often futile, always destructive—to control nature. As Carson (and others) saw it, pesticides were the means to controlling nature. Indeed, at an early point in Carson's writing of the book, the editor of Houghton Mifflin, Paul Brooks, suggested that the volume should be titled *The Control of Nature*, and for a short time this was its working title. By 1959, the working title Carson proposed was *Man Against the Earth* (Lear, 2009, p. 324).[1] In the end, she used neither title, but this general idea turned up again as the shout line on the jacket cover of the first edition of *Silent Spring*: "The author of *The Sea Around Us* and *The Edge of the Sea* questions our attempt to control the natural world around us!"

In *Silent Spring*, Carson questioned much of the received wisdom of her era. She fingered science, the military, industry, and government agencies as the parties most responsible for the ecocide she was witnessing. She challenged notions of what constituted "progress." She didn't share the boosterism of the 1950s and 1960s for atomic energy and "the bomb." She was a woman outside her culture in many ways, and this gave her a view from afar.

Carson, herself, is explicit about her larger frame of reference, and one could easily read *Silent Spring* in its entirety as a polemic against the human hubris of "control." Indeed, she ends her book with a warning and a lament that in the name of controlling nature, we will destroy it:

> The "control of nature" is a phrase conceived in arrogance, born of the Neanderthal age of biology and philosophy, when it was supposed that nature exists for the convenience of man. The concepts and practices of applied entomology for the most part date from that Stone Age of science. It is our alarming misfortune that so primitive a science has armed itself with the most modern and terrible weapons, and that in turning them against the insects it has also turned them against the earth.
>
> (pp. 261–262)

Carson, here, is making three critical points; foundational themes that weave throughout *Silent Spring*: first, that an impulse of human mastery and control underlies specific campaigns—whether of fire ant eradication or mosquito control—and that what's really going on is, at its root, an attempt to control nature; second, that controlling nature is an abhorrent, old-fashioned, "stone age" approach to human relations to the environment; and third, that science, in its efforts of control, now allows people to deploy fearsome weapons that threaten the entire earth, never available or imagined in earlier eras.

Throughout *Silent Spring*, Carson rails against the destruction caused by "man's" arrogant efforts to control nature. Indeed, the whole point of pesticides is to "control" something—insects, or weeds, or unwanted species. Thus, in the most immediate sense, *Silent Spring* is entirely about efforts to "control." Carson, as we will see in the next chapter, had a great deal to say about the ineffectual and dangerous outcomes of specific control programs. But at the same time, Carson frames *Silent Spring* as a critique about "control" in the big-picture sense. She is both alarmed and distressed that the new chemical era is aimed first and foremost towards the goal of the complete conquest of nature. In pursuit of that deadly goal, "man" "has written a depressing record of destruction, directed not only against the earth he inhabits but against the life that shares it with him" (p. 83).

Carson emphasized this theme again in several interviews after publication of *Silent Spring*, most explicitly in a 1963 *CBS Reports* interview:

> We still talk in terms of conquest. We still haven't become mature enough to think of ourselves as only a very tiny part of a vast and incredible universe. Now I truly believe that we in this generation must come to terms with nature . . . we're challenged, as mankind has never been challenged before, to prove our maturity and our mastery, not of nature but of ourselves.
>
> (cited in Lear, 2009, p. 450)

Science

Historians of science typically identify the European Renaissance (not the "stone age," a rhetorical flourish on Carson's part) as the era when both the ideology and the large-scale human capacity to control nature emerged. Carolyn Merchant (1980) broke fresh analytical ground when she identified the emergence of "modern" science in the sixteenth and seventeenth centuries as the pivotal shift from considering nature as alive and a force unto itself, to a rendering of nature as an object to be subjugated and controlled through the superior power of science and technology. For several centuries prior to the emergence of modern Western science, the cosmos was thought of as a living organism with a body, soul and spirit; the earth was alive, a nurturing mother. What we, in retrospect, call the "Scientific Revolution" changed all that. In the view of modern science, the dominant metaphor for nature became a mechanistic one: nature became an assemblage of atoms and parts, all of which could be—should be—known and controlled by "man."

In Merchant's analysis, science, with its modernist project of dominating nature, was a primary force in producing ecological crisis:

> For most of human history, nature had the upper hand over human beings, and humans fatalistically accepted the hand that nature dealt. People lived at the mercy of nature's storms, droughts, frosts, and famines. They accepted fate while propitiating nature with gifts, sacrifices, and prayer (often within hierarchical human relationships). Failed harvests, famines, and droughts were considered God's, or the Great Spirit's, way of blaming human beings for acting in an unethical way.
>
> Only in the last few centuries have technologies and attitudes of domination stemming from the Scientific Revolution turned the tables, enabling humans to threaten nature with deforestation and desertification, chemical pollution, destruction of habitats and species, nuclear fallout, and ozone depletion. Through mechanistic science, technology, capitalism, and the Baconian hubris that the human race should have dominion over the entire universe, humanity has gained an increasing ability to destroy nature.
>
> (Merchant, 2010, p. 3)

It was Baconian science, in particular, that developed and proclaimed a program for the domination of nature. The goal of modern science as shaped by Francis Bacon (1561–1626) and his contemporaries, (but Bacon particularly so), was to achieve complete knowledge of natural processes in order to gain mastery over them.

In the great struggle over how to conceptualize nature and human relationships to it—sensate or insensate, mother or object of inquisition, mysterious force or predictable laws, awe or reason—Bacon clearly won. The rationalist worldview of modernist science has indisputably prevailed.

To our collective misfortune, many would say. The German philosopher Max Horkheimer prefigured both Carson's and Merchant's analysis in 1947 with his extended argument that in an era of formalized reason, nature "has been stripped of all intrinsic value or meaning" (Horkheimer, 1985, p. 101). Horkheimer continues:

> The disease of reason is that reason was born from man's urge to dominate nature . . . One might say that the collective madness that ranges today, from the concentration camps to the seemingly most harmless mass-culture reactions, was already present in germ in primitive objectivization [sic], in the first man's calculating contemplation of the world as prey.
>
> (p. 176)

Much of contemporary environmentalism, certainly of environmental ethics, focuses on repairing the rip in the ecological fabric between humans and "nature" that scientific rationality, in tandem with capitalist production, has wrought (see, for example, Donovan, 1990; Leiss, 1972, 2007; Lovelock, 1979; McKibben, 1990; Merchant, 2003; Mies and Shiva, 1993; Oelschlaeger, 1993; Shiva, 1988; Taylor, 1986; Warren, 2000).

Many contemporary historians, philosophers, and environmentalists echo Horkheimer's further view that "[t]he history of man's efforts to subjugate nature is also the history of man's subjugation by man" (Horkheimer, 1985, p. 105). Collective domination over nature is matched at every stage by a comparably heightened domination by *some* people over others (Leiss, 2007; Pattberg, 2007).

Feminists have explicated the gender politics of this assessment. Merchant argued, for example, that the devaluation of *women*, long identified with nature, was particularly and specifically integral to the production of the emerging modernist scientific project. Nature, for nearly everyone in the Renaissance and Scientific Revolution, was female. More than a metaphor, nature was viewed, literally, as female—typically a nurturing mother. As a living being, Nature had a body, soul, and spirit; Nature personified had breasts, a bosom, and a womb, as well as circulatory, reproductive, and elimination systems (Merchant, 2010, p. 2).

As part of the modernist project, Merchant argues, control of nature was inextricably tied to men's control of women—metaphorically and literally. Bacon's scientific quest was to "wrest secrets from Nature's grasp" and to reveal the "secrets locked in Nature's bosom." Bacon talked of dominating and enslaving Nature, hounding her, and interrogating her into giving up her secrets (Merchant, 2008, p. 754). In the view of many analysts, this is not just rhetoric.

Recent feminist environmental analysis makes clear that the association of women with nature—and men's linked domination of both—is not only a seventeenth-century artifact. For example, a large corpus of writings on the sexualized representations of associations between animals and women (see Adams, 1990; Donovan, 1990; Emel, 1995); Vandana Shiva's work on contemporary oppressions of women and environment (1988, 1993); Val Plumwood's (1993) critiques of the "standpoint of mastery"; and my own work on masculinized structures of environmental agency (Seager, 1993a) among many others, extends and deepens Merchant's analysis of the origins of this ideology of dual dominance.

The masculinized domination of nature and, symbiotically, of women, is inextricable from the masculinized structure of modern science. To the extent that "men of reason" structured modern science in their own image as a project to wrest control from a feminized nature, then it follows that women would be placed largely outside the enterprise of science. Feminist historians and philosophers of science, such as Donna Haraway, Sandra Harding, and Evelyn Fox Keller, have contributed important analyses of the ways in which the standpoints of modern science exclude women or frame women as "other." The assumed and structured incompatibility of women and science—and between women and scientific rationality—continues to have enormous salience (Noble, 1991).[2] As it did in Rachel Carson's own life.

Carolyn Merchant and scholars of science who have followed in her footsteps not only implicate mechanistic science in creating the most pressing ecological problems of our day, they dare to suggest that women were as much the victims as the beneficiaries of the progress of science. Merchant's analysis, at its core, throws into doubt the "grand narratives" of science and progress, and questions the previously unexamined ways that modern science is assumed to have manufactured "progress":

> The notion of a "Scientific Revolution" in the sixteenth and seventeenth centuries is part of a larger mainstream narrative of Western culture that has propelled science, technology, and capitalism's efforts to "master" nature—a narrative into which most Westerners have unconsciously been socialized and within which we ourselves have become actors in a storyline of upward progress.
>
> (Merchant, 2006, p. 517)

Two decades before Carolyn Merchant, Carson, too, was questioning the nature of "progress" and asking "big questions" about the role of science in constructing a false narrative of what constituted progress. (However, Carson did not include any gender analysis in her work, nor did she indicate any familiarity with the then-nascent feminist movement and analysis emerging from contemporary writers such as Betty Friedan, whose *Feminine Mystique* was published a year after *Silent Spring*.)

The absence of feminist analysis aside, throughout *Silent Spring*, Carson laments the high price of the "modern way of life." Carson is amazed that we have brought death-stalking hazards into our world in the name of modernity. She expresses amazement that in the name of making "man's" life "easier," we are prepared to threaten all life on the planet, and to embrace the routine use of chemicals as a normal part of daily life and economy.

But Carson doesn't just lament, nor is she satisfied with a passive analysis that starts and ends with something as diffuse as blaming "our way of life." One of the reasons why *Silent Spring* was so controversial (and remains so) was that Carson identifies *specific* processes that produce consensus and stifle dissent about what is an acceptable ecological price. Further, she points to specific agents of authority and power who propel and profit from "our way of life." She fingers industry, the military, government agencies, and the structure of scientific knowledge.

Carson focuses much of her critical analysis on the processes of what Noam Chomsky, many years later, called "manufacturing consent." Carson asks pointedly and poignantly:

> Who has made the decision that sets in motion these chains of poisonings, this ever-widening wave of death? Who has placed in one pan of the scales the leaves that might have been eaten by the beetles and in the other the pitiful heaps of many-hued features, the lifeless remains of the birds that fell before the unselective bludgeon of insecticidal poisons? Who has decided—who has the *right* to decide—for the countless legions of people who were not consulted that the supreme value is a world without insects, even though it be also a sterile world ungraced by the curving wing of a bird in flight?
>
> (p. 118)

For Carson, these were not rhetorical questions. She really wanted to know, and she wants us to know. She believes that we have the *right* to know. Carson was ready to name names.

Science—industry—government collusion

Carson decries the role of science and scientists in setting the ideological frame and providing the means for the control of nature; she doesn't shy away from indicting science for the destructive pathway it had taken (Hynes, 1989, p. 7). And she is even *more* critical of what she sees as the increasingly cozy institutional and financial relationships between science and industry. She holds chemical industries directly accountable for promoting an ideology of the "habit of killing—the resort to 'eradicating' any creature that may annoy or inconvenience us" (p. 117). But she sounds a truly radical warning when she warns of the dangers of a public policy and science agenda driven by the pursuit of profit:

> It is . . . an era dominated by industry, in which the right to make a dollar at whatever cost is seldom challenged. When the public protests, confronted with some obvious evidence of damaging results of pesticide applications, it is fed little tranquilizing pills of half truth. We urgently need an end to these false assurances, to the sugar coating of unpalatable facts. It is the public that is being asked to assume the risks that the insect controllers calculate.
>
> (p. 23)

Little tranquilizing pills of half truth! Suggesting there should be limits to the pursuit of profits? This is an astonishingly forthright analysis to be presented to a country not even a decade beyond Red Scare McCarthyism. No wonder Carson's critics called her a communist!

Indeed, a century earlier, Karl Marx was among the first to decry the role of Baconian science as an endeavor aimed at subjugating nature to human interests, under the "ruse" of pure science. Marx twinned this with a critique of profit-seeking capital:

> Capital creates . . . the universal appropriation of nature as well as of the social bond itself . . . Nature becomes purely an object for humankind, purely a matter of utility; ceases to be recognized as a power for itself; and the theoretical discovery of its autonomous laws appears merely as a ruse so as to subject it under human needs, whether as an object of consumption or as a means of production.
>
> (Marx, 1973, p. 410)

Carson was far from being a Marxist; in terms of formal political affiliation, she was a Democrat (who worked for the election of John Kennedy, among other activities), and a fairly moderate one at that. Nor would she have appreciated all of Carolyn Merchant's critiques of science. But in many ways, Carson's arguments can be located along the spectrum of left-leaning thinkers—probably in the center of that spectrum, but nonetheless occupying an important place on it.

Despite her politically moderate inclinations, she was uncompromising in her critique of industry. She saved some of her fiercest criticisms for the cozy collusion she witnessed between industry and supposedly independent university scientists or government officials—the very people who should have provided a firewall against the practices of profit-seeking industries. She decried the influence of money in entomology that drew scientists away from research into non-chemical insect-control approaches and that kept them beholden to the chemical companies. Remarking that only about 2 percent of entomological scientists were then working in the field of biological controls, Carson is palpably pained that most insect scientists are more drawn to the "exciting" work in chemical control. Carson rhetorically asks "Why?" and in answering herself, points to the influence of funding. She remarks that chemical companies are pouring money into universities and research labs to support work on insecticides, while biological-control studies have no financial champions. There's no money to be made in biological control, she pointedly remarks.

She goes on to make the point that this cozy financial relationship undercuts the presumption of objectivity in the pursuit of science. She finds it mystifying that entomologists might ever be leading advocates of chemical control—an improbable position she attributes to the corrupting influence of the financial support of chemical companies. By the time Carson was writing *Silent Spring*, chemical companies had insinuated themselves into research institutes and academia, and were starting to produce privately funded science. The entomologists who promoted chemical controls were, Carson said, most likely supported by the chemical industry itself. Perhaps, Carson says ruefully, one couldn't expect them to "bite the hand that feeds them." But, she warns, this close relationship between industry funding and the research process means that conclusions that insecticides are "harmless" had little credibility. As science cozied up to industry, it undercut itself.

Carson's warning about the "science-industry" complex came at a distinctive moment in the midst of cultural shift in the way Americans were viewing large, powerful institutions—a shift prompted to some significant extent by President Dwight Eisenhower. It was in 1961, just as Carson would be finishing *Silent Spring*, that President Eisenhower (a retired general) surprised Americans in his farewell address with his now-famous warnings about the "unwarranted influence" of the "military-industrial complex":

This conjunction of an immense military establishment and a large arms industry is new in the American experience. The total influence—economic, political, even spiritual—is felt in every city, every Statehouse, every office of the Federal government. We recognize the imperative need for this development. Yet we must not fail to comprehend its grave implications. Our toil, resources and livelihood are all involved; so is the very structure of our society. In the councils of government, we must guard against the acquisition of unwarranted influence, whether sought or unsought, by the military-industrial complex. The potential for the disastrous rise of misplaced power exists and will persist.

(Eisenhower, 1961)

Eisenhower, like Carson, believed that the best defense against such unwarranted influence was an informed citizenry: "Only an alert and knowledgeable citizenry can compel the proper meshing of the huge industrial and military machinery of defense with our peaceful methods and goals, so that security and liberty may prosper together," he went on to say. Carson, too, believes that the responsibility to be informed—to know what was being done in our name—rests with those who held the reins of power *and also* with ordinary citizens. "We" as a citizenry, she says, have privileged the role of poison and poisoners, and allowed their ideology to prevail. She answers her own question, above, of "Who has made the decision that sets in motion these chains of poisonings . . . Who has decided . . ." with this sobering assessment:

> The decision is that of the authoritarian temporarily entrusted with power; he has made it during a moment of inattention by [the] millions to whom beauty and the ordered world of nature still have a meaning that is deep and imperative.
>
> (p. 118)

The *authoritarianism* is located elsewhere, in the institutions she critiques; but the *inattention* that allows this authoritarian to rule is *ours*, each of ours. This is an interesting post-World War II indictment, as the world was still echoing with unanswered questions about how the atrocities of that war, including mass genocides and holocausts, at the hands of authoritarians, could have been committed—in full view, and yet somehow not fully regarded.

However, at the same time that she holds each of us accountable for our "inattention", Carson understands that mere citizens cannot be fully expected to understand the complexities of the environmental effects of pesticides—indeed, Carson's point is precisely that many effects are unpredictable or not fully understood or, worse, are intentionally obscured. She understands that soft-sell marketing and clever persuasions could easily sway the average person.

Carson is thoroughly a modernist: she believes that there are "facts" that could be discovered and revealed, but that vested interests stand in the way of fact-finding. Carson believes that the public has a *right* to know what is going on, as well as having an *obligation* to know, but she understands that "the public" can only make informed choices if indeed they are informed by impartial expertise, not by experts who are reflecting vested interests.

Rather than holding individual citizens to account, Carson is searching for the "reliable narrator"—which is why she is so ferocious in her denunciations of government agencies that, in her view, shirk their responsibility to be neutral arbiters of truth. Entomologists in the thrall of chemical control programs are, in her estimation, particularly unreliable narrators. Entomologists working for chemical companies (or under their funding, directly or indirectly) could not be expected, Carson says, to honestly explore or expose the undesirable effects of chemical control. Carson is adamant that the public needs the judgment of unbiased observers who are not beholden to the chemical companies. But where to find those unbiased judges, she asks?

Carson laments that the modern structure of scientific knowledge, in which specialists know little of the "big picture" of their subject, works against the interest of comprehensive knowledge. Extreme specialization, Carson suggests, means that very few scientists have a "big picture" grasp of problems—each specialist understands his or her own small piece of the puzzle, but fewer and fewer scientists have a wholistic vision. Further, she understands that ordinary people are often confounded by conflicting advice from specialists. Carson understands that citizens, who might themselves not be particularly scientifically literate, are pulled between competing specialists. On the question of the extent of wildlife losses from pesticide exposures, for example, she explains:

> On the one hand conservationists and wildlife biologists assert that the losses have been severe and in some cases even catastrophic. On the other hand, the control agencies tend to deny flatly and categorically that such losses have occurred, or that they are of any importance if they have. Which view are we to accept?
> (p. 83)

Part of Carson's answer to this dilemma is what we would call today "citizen science." Carson says, more or less, that individuals should be attentive to what they see happening in their own homes and backyards—and that they can and should trust their own senses and their own observations. Carson wants to open up science, to knock it off its isolationist plinth. Carson believes that scientific findings should be understandable to a wide audience, and that scientific work should be open to public interrogation. She, herself, was practicing "democratized" science through her own writings. Carson's insistence that the directions and practices of science and technology could be open to public debate, input, and accountability was then—and is now—a challenge to the most cherished paradigm of science as a domain of a specialized few. We will return in Chapter 5 to her views on citizen science and the paradigmatic shift she was advancing through these views.

What is less remembered about Eisenhower's 1961 speech was that he warned, also, about the influence of money and vested interests in scientific research:

> Today, the solitary inventor, tinkering in his shop, has been overshadowed by task forces of scientists in laboratories and testing fields. In the same fashion, the free university, historically the fountainhead of free ideas and scientific discovery, has experienced a revolution in the conduct of research.
>
> Partly because of the huge costs involved, a government contract becomes virtually a substitute for intellectual curiosity. For every old blackboard there are now hundreds of new electronic computers. The prospect of domination of the nation's scholars by

Federal employment, project allocations, and the power of money is ever present—and is gravely to be regarded.

Yet, in holding scientific research and discovery in respect, as we should, we must also be alert to the equal and opposite danger that public policy could itself become the captive of a scientific-technological elite.

(Eisenhower, 1961)

The speech by Eisenhower—an Army general and a president who relied heavily on the military as a tool of statecraft—warning about the military-industrial complex, catalyzed a new awareness and wariness about vested interests. Carson's concerns about interlocking institutional relationships were less easy to dismiss in the wake of Eisenhower's warnings.

Post-*Silent Spring*, Carson's remarks about industry collusion with science became even sharper still. In a 1962 speech to the Women's National Press Club, she repeatedly warned against the corrupting influence of chemical companies funding basic science, and ended with a rousing denunciation of the "gods of profit and production":

A penetrating observer of social problems has pointed out recently that whereas wealthy families once were the chief benefactors of the Universities, now industry has taken over this role. Support of education is something no one quarrels with—but this need not blind us to the fact that research supported by pesticide manufacturers is not likely to be directed at discovering facts indicating unfavorable effects of pesticides. Such a liaison between science and industry is a growing phenomenon, seen in other areas as well. The AMA [American Medical Association], through its newspaper, has just referred physicians to a pesticide trade association for information to help them answer patients' questions about the effects of pesticides on man . . . We see scientific societies acknowledging as "sustaining associates" a dozen or more giants of a related industry . . . What does it mean when we see a committee set up to make a supposedly impartial review of a situation, and then discover that the committee is affiliated with the very industry whose profits are at stake? . . .

> Is industry becoming a screen through which facts must be filtered, so that the hard, uncomfortable truths are kept back and only the harmless morsels allowed to filter through? I know that many thoughtful scientists are deeply disturbed that their organizations are becoming fronts for industry. More than one scientist has raised a disturbing question—whether a spirit of Lysenkoism may be developing in America today—the philosophy that perverted and destroyed the science of genetics in Russia and even infiltrated all of that nation's agricultural sciences. But here the tailoring, the screening of basic truth, is done, not to suit a party line, but to accommodate to the short-term gain, to serve the gods of profit and production.
>
> (Carson, 1998b, pp. 208–210)

The suggestion that "Lysenkoism" was emerging in America would have shocked Carson's 1962 audience, immersed, as it was, in the grip of Cold War fear and revulsion of the Soviet Union. Lysenko was a Soviet agronomist who had enormous influence over food and agricultural policy in Stalin's Russia. His idiosyncratic views of genetics and crop productivity were imposed on the entire agricultural production chain in the Soviet Union—with disastrous consequences. Scientific dissent from Lysenko's theories was outlawed in 1948, and he ruled the biological sciences dictatorially. The term "Lysenkoism" thus has come to connote a corrupted scientific approach that doesn't necessarily search for "truth," but, rather, searches for evidence to support predetermined conclusions that are shaped by ideological predilections. For Carson to worry aloud about the emergence of a Lysenkoist-like distortion of American science (skewed not to hew to the line of party politics, in this case, but distorted by the pursuit of profit and corporate interests) was a shockingly stern warning from one of the best-known scientists of the time.

In Chapter 10 of *Silent Spring*, "Indiscriminately from the Skies," Carson describes two disastrously destructive aerial spraying programs—one against gypsy moths, and the other to "eradicate" (a chilling word if ever there was one) fire ants. Carson describes at great length the collateral damage from these reckless spraying programs, their utter failure in meeting original objectives, and the obstinacy of officials in the Department of Agriculture in the face of mounting opposition to spraying, and growing evidence of the damage wrought by these programs. Both programs, she argues, were based on "gross exaggeration of the need for control" (p. 142). She alludes to the likelihood—but never quite definitively says—that pesticide manufacturers looking for new markets concocted the sudden "need" for these spraying programs. Carson is clearly suspicious of the suddenness of the new programs designed to attack insects that had, to that point, not been seen as major pests or priorities for control. Carson doesn't unravel the trail of events that lead to these suddenly urgent campaigns, but, rather, cites an unnamed trade journal bragging, as the fire ant program got underway, that US pesticide makers had tapped a "sales bonanza" (p. 147) in the increasing numbers of pest elimination programs conducted by the US Department of Agriculture. Carson wryly notes that "Never has any pesticide program been so thoroughly and deservedly damned by practically everyone except the beneficiaries of this 'sudden bonanza'" (p. 147).

In many of her post-*Silent Spring* lectures, it seems that Carson felt more free to draw attention to the profit motive that was, in her view, driving the proliferation—and redundancy—of pesticides. In her 1963 testimony before a Congressional committee, she argued that regulators should impose a "needs test" before approving chemical production and use:

> It seems to me that our troubles are unnecessarily compounded by the fantastic number of chemical compounds in use as pesticides. As matters stand, it is quite impossible for research into the effect of these chemicals on the physical environment, on wildlife, and on man to keep pace with their introduction and use. It is hard to escape the conclusion that the great proliferation of new chemicals is dictated by the facts of competition within the industry rather than by actual need. I should like to see the day when new pesticides will be approved for use only when no existing chemical or other method will do the job.
>
> (Carson, 1963)

Many of Carson's critics understood that the subtext (and not very "sub" at that) of *Silent Spring* was a critique of the pesticide industry's profit-maximizing practices and contrived carelessness in the name of progress. So did her admirers. Loren Eiseley, the influential science writer, highlighted this theme in his review in *The Saturday Review*: "[*Silent Spring*] is a devastating, heavily documented, relentless attack upon human carelessness, greed and irresponsibility" (p. 18). A *New York Times* editorial published just prior to the book's publication, expressed the hope that *Silent Spring* might "arouse enough public concern to immunize government agencies against the blandishments of the hucksters" (cited in Lear, 1993, p. 36).

Militaries, militarism, and the atomic world

Carson was writing *Silent Spring* in the midst of a post-war technology and power high. The 1950s was a decade of unfettered American triumphalism. Boosterism about the triumphs of modern science was ubiquitous. The atomic bomb had won the war (or so it was said). The first patient received a mechanical heart. The polio vaccine was saving lives and lifting a terrifying threat from everyday life. A newfangled device called a "computer" was making waves. Middle-class households could suddenly be stocked with refrigerators, televisions, electric ovens, and a car in every garage; optimistic consumerism was the temper of the times. Commercial airline travel was booming and even ordinary people could imagine flying. The Soviets and the Americans were chasing each other into space. There seemed to be no limits to American ingenuity, American power, American know-how; the prevailing wisdom was that there *shouldn't* be limits.

Cathy Trost, author of an important exposé of the culture of chemical industries, describes the era in this way:

> There was little room in the 1950s for the advocates of the slow, thoughtful approach in any portion of life—business, science, or politics. The country was so firmly in control of itself and had tied technology so tightly to patriotism that to be skeptical . . . was to be a traitor. Nationwide publicity linking cigarettes to heart disease for the first time in 1954 was countered by advertisements that

pointed out reassuringly that "More Doctors Smoke Camels Than Any Other Cigarette." "The deadliest sin was to be controversial," observed William Manchester in describing a generation that wanted "the good, sensible life" and that was "proud to be conservative, prosperous, conformist and vigilant defenders of the American way of life." The largest group of college undergraduates were business majors, and industry leaders were lionized (General Motors president Harlow Curtice was *Time*'s Man of the Year in 1956). A free market, left to its own devices, was thought to be the most efficient path to productivity. In 1957 the Soviets simultaneously launched Sputnik 1 and the space race by taunting Americans with the specter of Russian superiority. Obeisance to technocracy took on patriotic as well as religious overtones.

The chemical industry was in its florescence, and its leaders spared no hyperbole in promoting it—and private enterprise in general—as the last line of defense against moral and economic collapse, world famine and Communist takeover.

(Trost, 1984, p. 33)

As the "American way of life" was being redefined in the Cold War that followed World War II, a significant part of that redefinition involved control over nature. This was not only deemed a necessary element of the American project, but, given the tremendous advances in science and technology, it seemed within reach. Starting with the 1930s Public Works Administration, Big Engineering marked the ascent towards the "American century": the Hoover Dam, the Tennessee Valley Authority engineering works, the start of the channelization of the Mississippi River. In the 1940s and 1950s, the pace of these large-scale works accelerated, and even bigger projects pushed forward: the conceptualization and start of construction for the interstate highway network; the compoundment and draining of the Everglades; the channelization of the Missouri River; the control of the Colorado River.[3]

The US military was the driving force behind much of this post-war, Cold War, enthusiasm for controlling nature. One of its branches—the Army Corps of Engineers—was integral to the biggest of the big civilian engineering projects (as it is still, to a large degree). The Corps, established by Thomas Jefferson in 1802, was given primary responsibility for flood control in the 1930s; since then, they have dammed, channeled, contained, drained, straightened, and boxed in the rivers of the United States with abandon. For most of its history, the Corps was unabashed about its mission to tame nature. The history of the Corps is interwoven with the nation-building, European-American frontier ethic of mighty men subduing a big land. The official history of the Corps, until recently, proudly reported that Corps engineers "were the pathfinders sent out by a determined government at Washington. They guided, surveyed, mapped and fought Indians and nature across the continent" (cited in Seager, 1993b). In 1970, the chief of the Corps explained to a journalist that "we cannot simply sit back and let nature take its course" (Drew, 1970, p. 53). Underscoring its reputation, a *Washington Post* reporter recently referred to the Corps as "the ground troops in America's war on nature" (Grunwald, 2006, p. 5). And the Corps didn't just manage waterways. Its engineering reach ranged from dams, to highways, to "managing" whole ecosystems such as the Everglades; everywhere it went, its goal was to tame, control, and master nature (O'Brien, 2007).

The Corps established an environmental division in the late 1960s, but had a hard time embracing the growing interest in ecological protection. Several speeches by leaders in the Corps in the late 1960s, reflect the persistence of the entrenched "let nothing stand in our way" militarized attitude that alarmed Carson a few years earlier. The Director of the Corps' Civil Works Division remarked to an audience in 1970: "This business of ecology. We're concerned, but people don't know enough about how to give good advice. You have to stand still and study life cycles [in ecological studies], and we don't have" (Drew, 1970, p. 61). In the same year, the deputy director of the same division advanced the "rational man" argument for progress:

> It is a fact that our nation is engaged in a struggle to survive its technology and its habits. It is a fact, too, that we are defiling our waters, polluting our air, littering our land, and infecting our soil and ourselves with the wastes which our civilization produces. These are serious problems, but we cannot permit ourselves to yield to an emotional impulse that would make their cure the central purpose of our society. Nor is there any reason why we should feel

guilty about the alterations which we have to make in the natural environment as we meet our water-related needs.

(cited in Drew, 1970, p. 61)

In the 1950s, as Carson was writing *Silent Spring*, the US military was feeling its oats. This was a military on the move, and nature had to bend to its wishes; the military didn't just flex its nature-bending might through the Corps. Indeed, in relation to other military programs, the Corps of Engineers shrinks in importance. The really big card that the US military was holding was atomic power. In the 1950s, the US military was one of the most privileged institutions in American society. Fresh off its World War II victory, and moving into the heart of the Cold War, the US military went from being a minor force, prior to the war, to being *the* preeminent institution leading the United States to global prominence and dominance. The atomic energy program was what made the US military a "big deal," globally speaking. And domestically.

The US military's atomic program represented a pinnacle of scientific and technological accomplishment. The general trajectory of its "success" is well known—from the first experimental test of an atomic bomb (the Trinity test in New Mexico in June 1945), to the August 6, 1945 uranium bomb dropped on Hiroshima, Japan, followed on August 9, 1945 by a plutonium bomb dropped on Nagasaki. The first thermonuclear (hydrogen) bomb was exploded on Eniwetok Atoll in the Pacific in 1952, with the largest explosion to date produced by another thermonuclear device on the Bikini Atoll in 1954. Between 1945 and 1963—the era of atmospheric testing—the US military conducted more than 200 above-ground nuclear tests, about half in the Pacific and half in the US at the Nevada test site; the Russians conducted about an equal number.[4] Russia, Great Britain and the United States moved their nuclear testing underground after signing the Limited Test Ban Treaty in 1963. France, which didn't sign the treaty, continued underwater tests in the Pacific until the mid-1990s.

The health and environmental consequences of these (and the later several- hundred underground tests) have been nothing short of catastrophic. It is not only the actual bomb testing that has wrought so much environmental damage. The entire nuclear chain of production—manufacturing sites, waste storage, component sites—

has proven to be deadly. For example, during World War II, a semi-desert area in south-central Washington state was chosen as the site for one of three atomic cities to be built by the US Army to support the atomic bomb project. The Hanford reservation, as the installation is known, supplied the plutonium for the 1945 atomic bomb test at Alamogordo, New Mexico, and for the bomb that a month later destroyed Nagasaki. The secrecy surrounding the production of the first atomic bombs and the early years of the nuclear weapons build-up also concealed the fact that radioactive by-products of Hanford plutonium contaminated a large part of the Pacific Northwest—and worse, that officials at the plant were aware of the contamination, and worse still, that some of it was deliberate.

Over the years, in their zeal to produce plutonium, Hanford's managers routinely allowed huge clouds of radioactive iodine, ruthenium, cesium, and other elements to be released from the processing plants' emission stacks. Liquid wastes were dumped directly into the Columbia River. Reports that were declassified in 1986, establish that pasturelands, crop lands, and forests hundreds of miles away were repeatedly contaminated; radioactive iodine is today present in the aquifers (the main water source for the region) under the Hanford reservation, and in farmers' wells across the Columbia River. Further, the reports give clear evidence that health specialists at Hanford recognized at the time the health risks of releasing so much radiation, but remained quiet.

One of the worst releases of radioactive material at Hanford was during a deliberate experiment in 1949. The Atomic Energy Commission (AEC), in charge of the plant at the time, and the US Army assumed that the Soviets were rushing to produce atomic bombs; further, they believed that the Soviets were using technology that would leave a measurable radioactive trace. They decided to test their assumptions in eastern Washington by creating radioactivity levels in the Hanford area similar to those that they presumed to exist near Soviet plants in order to see how easy it would be to identify the radioactive signal. The experiment, called "green run," released into the atmosphere some 5,500 curies of iodine 131, and a still-classified inventory of other fission products, secretly measured by the AEC, in a 200-by-40-mile plume. There was no public health warning. The government used the population around Hanford as guinea pigs, releasing radioactivity into the food, water, milk, and air, without consent or warning. (The nine reactors at Hanford are all now closed in response to the public exposé of safety hazards. But 60 million gallons of high-level radioactive waste remain stored "temporarily" at the site, and waste disposal ditches and lagoons remain full.)

Hanford is just one of dozens of casualty sites from the US nuclear program. Similar stories have been revealed about Rocky Flats (Colorado), the Savannah River site (South Carolina), Los Alamos National Laboratory (New Mexico), the Feed Materials Production Center (Ohio), among a dozen more (Seager, 1993a; Shulman, 1992; Schneider, 1991). Much remains classified about the nuclear program, but sufficient information about the health and environmental consequences of the nuclear program has been forced into the public domain that in 1990 the US government passed the "Radiation Exposure Compensation Act" (RECA). The US Department of Justice describes RECA in this way:[5]

> The Act presents an apology and monetary compensation to individuals who contracted certain cancers and other serious diseases:
>
> - following their exposure to radiation released during the atmospheric nuclear weapons tests, or
>
> - following their occupational exposure to radiation while employed in the uranium industry during the Cold War arsenal build-up.
>
> This unique statute was designed to serve as an expeditious, low-cost alternative to litigation. Notably, RECA does not require claimants to establish causation. Rather, claimants qualify for compensation by establishing the diagnosis of a listed compensable disease after working or residing in a designated location for a specific period of time. The Act provides compensation to individuals who contracted one of 27 medical conditions. It covers all states where uranium was mined and processed, as well as specified counties in Nevada, Utah, and Arizona, where significant fallout from the atmospheric nuclear testing was measured . . . RECA establishes lump sum compensation awards

for individuals who contracted specified diseases in three defined populations:

- Uranium miners, millers, and ore transporters—$100,000;
- "Onsite participants" at atmospheric nuclear weapons tests—$75,000; and
- Individuals who lived downwind of the Nevada Test Site ("downwinders")—$50,000.

When Carson was writing *Silent Spring* in the late 1950s and early 1960s, the most disastrous health and environmental consequences of the superpowers' nuclear programs were not yet known. But some activists and scientists were starting to raise alarms. Prominent public intellectuals, among them many scientists, gathered at the "Pugwash" meeting in 1957[6] in response to a Manifesto issued in 1955 by Bertrand Russell and Albert Einstein that called on scientists of all political persuasions to assemble to discuss the threat posed to civilization by thermonuclear weapons. The Manifesto was also signed by Max Born, Percy Bridgman, Leopold Infeld, Frederic Joliot-Curie, Herman Muller,[7] Linus Pauling, Cecil Powell, Joseph Rotblat, and Hideki Yukawa.

In the late 1950s, the St. Louis Committee for Nuclear Information, organized by Louise and Eric Reiss and Barry Commoner, among others, (and based on a prior St. Louis women's campaign for pure milk), helped to create both scientific knowledge and public awareness around the health dangers of radioactivity. "Radiological health protection," as the government would come to call it, was becoming such a public concern that in 1959 President Eisenhower established the Federal Radiation Council to provide scientific assessments of the available evidence on health effects of radiation exposure from natural, medical, and weapons testing sources. Its first report, issued in 1961, seriously underestimated the dangers and extent of public exposure, but the founding of this Council was an important acknowledgement of a dramatically growing problem.[8]

The Women's Strike for Peace movement in the early 1960s, propelled even further attention to weapons proliferation and to dangers from radiation, including the danger of strontium-90 in the milk supply of the nation. The nationwide strike of women in 1961 over weapons proliferation and radiation fallout shocked the country and drew more attention to the mounting problems of radioactive releases (Swerdlow, 1993).

Carson, alarmed by radiation releases and, indeed, by the whole nuclear enterprise, was an unwavering critic of the Cold War and its atomic age. Even though site-specific problems such as Hanford were not yet fully comprehended, due mostly to government secrecy, there were dozens of examples of malfeasance, accidents, negligence, and recklessness with highly lethal nuclear materials about which Carson and her contemporaries *did* know. One of the most notorious was the "Lucky Dragon" catastrophe. On March 1, 1954, the 23 crew members of the Japanese tuna fishing boat "Daigo Fukuryu Maru" (the "Lucky Dragon"), on that day fishing in the North Pacific, were enveloped for several hours in a white, ashy fog of "snow." Within hours, the fishermen began to get sick. After returning to Japan, several of the fishermen spent months in hospital, and one died. The "snow" that had enveloped their boat was nuclear fallout from the experimental US hydrogen bomb detonation on Bikini atoll. Misjudging the strength of the explosion—1,000 times stronger than Hiroshima—the US government didn't provide sufficient warning to boats in the area (nor to locally stationed US personnel, nor to Micronesian islanders, also caught in the fallout). Marking the 58th anniversary of the Lucky Dragon incident, *The Japan Times* revisited the story this way in 2012:

> [Oishi, one of the fishermen] writes: "A yellow flash poured through the porthole. Wondering what had happened, I jumped up from the bunk near the door, ran out on deck and was astonished. Bridge, sky and sea burst into view, painted in flaming sunset colors . . ."
> What Oishi saw was the first US test of a dry-fuel thermonuclear device, code-named "Castle Bravo." At 15 megatons, it was the largest nuclear test ever conducted by the US, and remains the fifth-largest nuclear explosion in history. It was also, in a sense, an accident. A theoretical error by the bomb's designers meant that the explosion that actually occurred was 2½ times more powerful than intended. It was, in fact, the biggest-ever explosion made by

humankind, and was up to 1,000 times more powerful than the one that had razed Hiroshima nine years before.

Lucky Dragon wasn't damaged by the blast or its shock wave, but several hours later white, radioactive dust from atomized coral that had surged up to the edge of the atmosphere in an enormous plume began raining down on the Lucky Dragon and all aboard.

As Oishi writes: "The top of the cloud spread over us. . . Two hours passed . . . white particles were falling on us, just like sleet. The white particles penetrated mercilessly—eyes, nose, ears, mouth. We had no sense that it was dangerous." While the fallout continued to rain down, the crew spent six hours pulling in the lines before setting course for home.

(*The Japan Times*, 2012)

In her chapter on the human health effects of exposure to synthetic chemicals (Chapter 14, "One in Every Four"), Carson recounts dozens of documented deaths from pesticide exposure, including one in which she draws a direct parallel between fallout from pesticides and from radiation, using the Lucky Dragon story to underscore the threat and the similitude. Carson tells the story of a Swedish farmer (pp. 204–205) who, like the Japanese fisherman, was a healthy young man working his land using modern farming techniques—including DDT and benzene hexachloride. As he was distributing the 60 pounds of chemicals on his acreage, winds pushed the dust back on the farmer and he was briefly enveloped in a cloud of pesticides. Within hours he felt tired; within days he was seriously ill. The Swedish farmer spiraled down into ever more serious illness and died after three months, his bone marrow almost entirely destroyed.

Carson was acutely worried about the threat of wholesale poisoning of people and ecosystems posed by the atomic age. In the last public speech she gave, in 1963 at the annual meeting of the Kaiser Foundation Hospitals, Carson talked at length about the poisoning of the world's oceans by the dumping of radioactive wastes at sea. In that speech, she focused in considerable detail on the transport of radioactive wastes through the marine ecosystem and food system. She observed that radioactive wastes dumped at sea— or radioactive materials falling on oceans after bomb tests—could possibly be considered "safe" if they stayed in one place, but that in the dynamic ecosystem of the world's oceans this would be impossible. Not only are radioactive materials dispersed in the marine environment by currents, waves, and winds, but marine organisms themselves transport radiation. In Carson's explanation of marine dynamics to the 1963 audience, one sees the naturalist author of *The Edge of the Sea* and *The Sea Around Us* at work:

> Marine organisms bring about a marked distribution, both vertical and horizontal, of the radioactive contaminants. As the plankton make regular migrations, sinking into deep water in the daytime and rising to the surface at night, with the organisms go the radioisotopes they have absorbed, or that may adhere to them. As a result, the contaminants are made available to other organisms in new areas; and as they are taken up by larger, more active animals, they are subject to transport over long horizontal distances; migrating fishes, seals and whales may distribute radioactive materials far beyond their point of origin. It is surprising that so little thought seems to have been given to the biological cycling of materials in one of the most crucial problems of our time: the understanding of the true hazards of radiation and fallout.
> (Carson, 1998b, pp. 236–237)

This leads her to muse on our collective unwillingness to make provision or policy around the understanding that environmental contaminants might pose a systemic threat to environments and all life, including humans. Carson doesn't understand the complacency with which chemicals are greeted. In her 1963 speech to the Kaiser Foundation Hospitals, she went on to remark that:

> It may be admitted freely, for example, that an agricultural chemical entering a river could kill thousands of fish; but it will be denied that this chemical could do any harm to the person who might drink the water. Reports of the decimation of whole populations of birds are shrugged off with the thought that it can't happen to us.
> (Carson, 1998b, p. 244)

Carson was so attentive to the militarized nuclear threat, that the first chemical she mentions in *Silent Spring* is not a pesticide, but strontium-90, a by-product of nuclear explosions. She writes in her opening chapter: "[strontium-90] released through nuclear explosions into the air, comes to earth in rain or drifts down as fallout, lodges in soil, enters into the grass or corn or wheat grown there, and in time takes up its abode in the bones of a human being, there to remain until his death" (p. 16). In the next sentence, she moves seamlessly to make the comparison with pesticides, which also fall to earth invisibly and initiate a silent sequence of illness and death.

In highlighting strontium-90 in *Silent Spring*, Carson had her finger on the public pulse. In 1961, the St. Louis Committee (see above) issued its first report of its now-famous study of baby teeth tracing strontium-90 uptake in humans. Strontium-90 (released by aboveground nuclear weapons testing) is rapidly absorbed in calcium in the human body—i.e., bones and teeth. In a stroke of brilliance, the St Louis Committee determined that strontium-90 would be easily detected in the baby teeth shed by growing children. The team sent baby-teeth collection teams to schools in St. Louis and organized a mail-in campaign, ultimately collecting over 300,000 teeth before the research ended in 1970. Preliminary results published by the team in *Science* in November 1961, revealed that levels of strontium-90 had risen steadily in children born during the period of heaviest aboveground nuclear testing—the 1950s—with those born later in the decade showing the most increased levels (Reiss, 1961).[9] The 1961 St. Louis Committee report was widely disseminated and discussed; fallout was on Americans' minds in the early 1960s.

Throughout *Silent Spring*, Carson drew attention to the silent, similar, mechanisms of both pesticides and radiation. Indeed, it's hard for a reader to tell whether the "white granular powder" (p. 14) that signifies the evil that is visited on her fabled town in Chapter 1 is radiation or pesticide residue; it could be either, and that's, perhaps, her point. Further, in Carson's view, it's not just that pesticides and radiation have similar mechanisms or cause similar damage, it's that they are both products of humans' reckless over-reach and the untrammeled use of powers beyond our moral capacity—and, indeed, beyond our control. In her opening chapter, immediately following the fable of the town struck down, Carson makes this plain. It is only now, in our modern era, Carson says, that humans have acquired the power to actually alter the nature of the environment that surrounds us—and to do so permanently. And with radiation and pesticides, the character of human interference with nature has shifted from a force of assault to a force of fatal evil, changing both in magnitude and character:

> This pollution is for the most part irrecoverable; the chain of evil it initiates not only in the world that must support life but in the living tissues is for the most part irreversible. In this now universal contamination of the environment, *chemicals are the sinister and little-recognized partners of radiation* [emphasis added] in changing the very nature of the world – the very nature of its life.
>
> (pp. 16–17)

Carson goes on to detail the similar mechanisms of strontium-90 and of pesticides. She describes radioactive fallout lodging in the soil, being taken up into grasses and crops, and, sinisterly, over time insinuating itself into human bones and bodies. Chemical exposures, Carson writes, follow this same, slow, deliberative chain of poisoning. Chemicals pass from one to another in an accumulating sequence of poisoning. Worse, Carson warns, these chemicals can be transported by water and wind far from where they were first deposited. No one knows quite where they will turn up, especially once they get into the underground water system. Mysteriously, chemical transformations occur, and one chemical form can take quite another shape; Carson quotes Albert Schweitzer's observation that "man can hardly even recognize the devils of his own creation" (p. 17).

Carson elaborates the point that "man" has created an unprecedented biological and cultural challenge—the speed with which humans are creating and embracing new poisonous chemicals reflects "the impetuous and heedless pace of man rather than the deliberate pace of nature" (p. 17). The man-made compounds of radioactivity and synthetic chemicals may appear to have natural analogues—radiation, for example, exists in nature—but these new materials have no natural counterparts. And, Carson warns, the vast scale on which these materials are distributed, and the speed with which they are introduced into nature, allow no time for biological adjustment or human evaluation.

Carson saw considerable similarity between the ideology of the development and use of radiation and the development of synthetic chemicals, and in their similar health and environmental consequences; they were the evil twins of her age. Carson made the unmistakable argument that atomic power and pesticides together represented paramount threats to all life on the planet—indeed to the very existence of life:

> Along with the possibility of the extinction of mankind by nuclear war, the central problem of our age has therefore become the contamination of man's total environment with such substances of incredible potential for harm—substances that accumulate in the tissues of plants and animals and even penetrate the germ cells to shatter or alter the very material of heredity upon which the shape of the future depends.
>
> (p. 18)

To Carson, the parallels between nuclear radiation and pesticides were striking: both posed unseen threats that moved through ecosystems as silent killers; both accumulate in human bodies over several years before their deadly effects are evident; both were alarming new artifices, both developed and unleashed by military hubris. She was alarmed that while there was growing public concern about radiation, there seemed much less interest in the chemical assault: "The fact that chemicals may play a [similar] role . . . has scarcely dawned on the public mind, nor on the minds of most medical or scientific workers" (pp. 189–190). Linda Lear remarks on the parallel that, to Carson, was unmistakably evident:

> While writing about the potentially deadly threat of one contaminant, Carson was acutely aware of its similarity to the type of deadly pollution that had gripped the public imagination [nuclear contamination]. In August 1945 *Time* had published pictures of the first atomic bomb explosion in Alamogordo, New Mexico, alongside a report announcing DDT as the ultimate weapon in the war on insects . . . The two products of wartime science were forever linked in discovery, destruction, and debate.
>
> (Lear, 2009, p. 374)

As we see later, the genetic mutations produced both by radiation and pesticides were of particular concern to Carson.

In Carson's estimation, both nuclear power and pesticide power derived from an enormous hubris and arrogance of "man." She saw that both gave humans enormous power over nature—which they were misusing with great alacrity. As Patricia Hynes notes, "[Carson] summed it up as a shift in the balance of power between men and nature, wrought by technology developed for World War II, and afterwards billed as mid-twentieth century progress to legitimate its postwar use in society" (Hynes, 1989, p. 7).

In *Silent Spring*, Carson highlighted the role of the US military in another episode of catastrophic pollution that, by the early 1960s as she was finishing the book, had become a public scandal: the massive pollution from the Rocky Mountain Arsenal near Denver, Colorado. The Arsenal, as Carson recounts, manufactured war materials starting in 1943. Shortly after this manufacturing began, farmers nearby started to report livestock deaths and odd livestock illnesses, crop losses, and human illnesses that at least some of the neighbors thought were related to the Arsenal.

What Carson doesn't say is that the Arsenal was manufacturing chemical weapons, including mustard gas, lewisite, and chlorine gas; in the early 1950s, in support of the Korean War effort, the Arsenal went on to manufacture phosphorous bombs, cluster bombs, and nerve gas. Carson picks up the story with the leasing of part of the Arsenal property in the early 1950s to private industry: the Julius Hyman & Company, bought by the Shell Chemical Company (a subsidiary of Shell Oil) in 1952, manufactured pesticides on the site. (Carson doesn't name the manufacturers, referring instead simply to "a private oil company" (p. 47).)

As illnesses and crop losses mounted, investigators in the late 1950s found massive pollution of drinking wells, irrigation systems, and groundwater in a several-mile radius from the site. For years, it turns out, the military operators as well as the private operators had dumped wastes into open evaporation ponds, unlined pits, and poorly-lined wells and pits. The full extent of the pollution—and of public outrage—would not be known for another 20 years; in the 1980s, it was declared as the "Superfund site" that was the most polluted place in the country.[10] But even by the late 1950s, enough was known about the problems at the Rocky Mountain Arsenal to draw Carson's attention. In *Silent Spring*, she focuses on the Arsenal to illustrate how easily chemicals are transported through groundwater and surface water systems. Carson alerts her readership to the reality that, because groundwater flows in interconnected systems, pesticides or contaminants added in one place will be transported through the entire system. Nature, Carson reminds us, doesn't operate in closed and separate compartments. From her earliest naturalist writings about the sea, Carson took great care to explore and reveal the reality of the interconnectedness of natural systems. For the general public of the early 1960s, the ecosystems idea that "everything is connected" was still novel.

To Carson, it was no coincidence that radioactive materials and pesticides were both products of the military. She is never directly critical of the military or of what we would today call "militarism," but she plainly places accountability for much environmental and health recklessness with the military, or, as Eisenhower would have it, with the military-industrial complex. In Chapter 3, "Elixirs of Death," in which Carson lays out the origins and basic chemical nature of insecticides, she identifies the military origins of the ubiquitous poisoning of humans, animals, and environment by synthetic chemicals. The creation of pesticides was literally a by-product of war. Insecticides were discovered as by-products of the laboratory development of chemical weaponry. It was a German scientist, Gerhard Schrader, who discovered the insecticidal properties of some of the chemical weapons then being tested by the German government. Building on Schrader's work, Carson recounts, the German government developed both nerve gases (which would shortly thereafter be used with deadly consequences) as well as insecticides.

DDT was catapulted into large-scale production, and then into civilian life, by the US military. It was not until the US military saw DDT's potential as a chemical weapon against typhus in Europe and malaria in the Pacific that it became a mass-produced chemical—at first, for the exclusive use of the military, and then, as the war was ending, DDT was being pushed into the civilian market as an agricultural and household insecticide.

In her narrative of the development of the practice of aerial spraying of pesticides, Carson notes that it was the availability of World War II surplus airplanes that made this possible:

> [Formerly, poisons] were kept in containers marked with skull and crossbones . . . With the development of the new organic insecticides and the abundance of surplus planes after the Second World War, all this was forgotten . . . they have amazingly become something to be showered down indiscriminately from the skies.
> (p. 141)

Throughout *Silent Spring*, Carson underscores the point that pesticides derived not only from an ideology of the "control" of nature, but, true to their military origins, represented an ideological proclivity towards outright war *on* nature. She introduces this theme within the first few pages of her book:

> [Pesticides] are used in man's war against nature. . . These sprays, dusts, and aerosols are now applied almost universally to farms, gardens, forests, and homes—nonselective chemicals that have the power to kill every insect, the "good" and the "bad," to still the song of birds and the leaping of fish in the streams, to coat the leaves with a deadly film, and to linger on in soil—all this though the intended target may be only a few weeds or insects. Can anyone believe it is possible to lay down such a barrage of poisons on the surface of the earth without making it unfit for all life? They should not be called "insecticides," but "biocides."
> (p. 18)

She continues her stark assessment, explaining that, once started, the process of developing and applying even more powerful chemicals spirals endlessly upwards driven by its own internal logic—and driven by the biological process of resistance. Insects quickly develop resistance to one chemical or the other, so the whole process must be continuously reinvented with ever-deadlier compounds. She warns that this is a battle where humans don't have the upper hand. The chemical war, Carson says, will never be "won," but the skirmishes and battles threaten all human, plant, and animal life.

She repeats this theme of human society conducting a "war on nature" throughout *Silent Spring*: "[of the 500 new chemicals introduced each year] among them are many that are used in man's *war against nature*" (p. 18); "DDT was hailed as a means ... of winning the *farmers' war against crop destroyers*" (p. 29); "the deadly chemicals that are being used in *our war against the insects*. What of our simultaneous *war against the weeds?*" (p. 41); "the *chemical war* [against the Japanese beetle] went on in succeeding years" (p. 91); "Yet at so fearful a risk, the farmers waged *their needless war on blackbirds*" (p. 118); "The [Agriculture] Department's *all-out chemical war* on the gypsy moth began on an ambitious scale" (p. 143).

And in perhaps her most compelling use of the metaphor, she frames the problem in a way that would resonate particularly with a readership on the rebound from the horrors of World War II: "The question is whether any civilization can wage relentless war on life without destroying itself, and without losing the right to be called civilized" (p. 95).

In one stunning paragraph, she invokes a backslide from peace to war (plowshares being beaten *back* into guns) and the terrible cost of the trivial pursuit of "the new":

> The chemical weed killers are a bright new toy ... they give a giddy sense of power over nature to those who wield them, and as for the long-range and less obvious effects—these are easily brushed aside as the baseless imaginings of pessimists. The "agricultural engineers" speak blithely of "chemical plowing" in a world that is urged to beat its plowshares into spray guns.
>
> (p. 69)

We might say Carson is previewing here the flip modern colloquialism about "boys with their toys."

Just as we can see the ways in which the development (and current practice, still) of science is "gendered," so too are militaries and engineering practices. The masculinist monopoly on militaries and of engineering is an important source of male power in contemporary society, as it was in the 1950s. Feminist technology studies detail some of the ways in which engineering and technology are highly masculinized endeavors—not only in practitioner profile (most engineers, for example, are men), but in the ideology and nature of the engineering and technology enterprises (see, for example, Balsamo, 1996; Cockburn, 1983, 1993; Hacker, 1989; Oldenziel, 1999; Seager, 1993b; Wajcman, 1991).

So are militaries (see Enloe, 2000, 2002). Put together—engineering prowess with military might—they create an almost-impenetrable masculine hegemony. Not only do they share characteristics of hegemonic masculinities, but militaries and engineering—to get back to Carson, here—are all about control. And it's a masculinized control. Once again, as with Bacon's science, with the thrall of fearsome powers of chemical assault on nature we can see the ideology of "man" (really, meaning "man") controlling nature. Carson didn't engage in gendered analysis of any kind, but one might map backwards to see elements of these analyses nascent in Carson's understanding of the state of the world.

Although Carson talks about the proliferation of pesticides and the several thousand brand names[11] they are sold under, she doesn't actually name any of the names. This was a missed opportunity—even a brief survey of contemporary commercial pesticides amplifies Carson's point of their war-like ideological roots. Pesticides today, as in Carson's time, are marketed to "appeal" to the impulse to control and conquer in ludicrously exaggerated ways:

A selection of commercial names of pesticides on the US market, 2012[12]

- ACHIEVE •ACTION •AIM •ALLEGIANCE •ALLY •AMBUSH
- AMMO • ANVIL • APOCALYPSE •ARSENAL •ASCEND •ASSERT
- ASSET •AUTHORITY FIRST •AVENGE •BARRAGE •BARRICADE
- BICEP II •BOUNDARY •BRAVO •BRAWL •BRAWL II •BRIGADE
- BROADSTRIKE •BULLET •CADET •CADRE •CAPTURE
- CHAMPION •CHARGER •CLINCHER •COBRA •COMMAND
- CONTAIN •CYCLONE •DISRUPT •DOMAIN •DUAL MAGNUM
- EMINENT EXPERT •ENFORCER •EXTREME •FALCON
- FIRESTORM •FIRSTSHOT •FORCE •FRONTIER •FRONTLINE
- FURY •FUSILADE •GOAL •GUARDSMAN •GUNSLINGER
- HARNESS • HAVOC • HI-YIELD KILLZALL •HINDER •HONCHO
- HONOR GUARD • HOT SHOT •IGNITE •IMPACT • INFANTRY 4L
- JAVELIN •JURY •LANDMASTER •LASSO •LEADER •LIBERTY

•LIGHTNING •MACHETE •MARKSMAN •MAVERICK •MEDAL •MUSTER •OUST •PAYLOAD •PENTAGON •PERMIT •PINNACLE •PONDMASTER •POUNCE •PROPEL •PROWL •PURSUIT •PURSUIT PLUS •PYTHON •QUASH •QUICK KILL •RAGE •RAMPAGE •RAPTOR •READYMASTER •RECOIL •RECRUIT •REFLEX •RELY •RESCUE •RESOLVE •RESPECT •REVENGE •REVOLVER •RODEO •ROUNDUP •SABER •SALVO •SAVAGE •SCEPTER •SCOPE •SCOUT X-TRA •SCYTHE •SHOCKWAVE •SHOTGUN •SLAY •SLEDGEHAMMER •SONAR •SPARTAN •SPIKE •SQUADRON •STEADFAST •STINGER •STOMP •STRONGARM •SUBDUE •SURGE •TALON •TENACITY • TOTAL KILL •TOP GUN •TOUCHDOWN •TOUGH GUY •TRIGGER •TRIPLE THREAT •TRIUMPH •TURBO •VALOR •VANQUISH •VERDICT •VOLLEY •WARRIOR •YIELD SHIELD

Crises of confidence

Post-war America was, in many ways, a brashly confident place. The United States emerged from World War II with one of the only intact industrial economies in the world; it was rapidly being propelled into global superpower status; the health and wealth of the nation and its people seemed more robust than ever; and American culture was starting to set the global norm. Carson was writing *Silent Spring* in an American context infused with the sense of American destiny being shaped, literally, by "big science," big engineering, and an all-encompassing military predominance—all wrapped in a thick cloak of secrecy. At the same time, Americans were encouraged to be paranoid about the security of their world, with Cold War fear of communism and the Soviet Union being whipped up by their government.

Nonetheless, there were cracks in the façade of the boisterous enthusiasm for the unfettered science/engineering/military-driven American path to modernity. Fallout (radioactive and otherwise) from the escalating superpower arms race was just one of the worries on the public agenda. Several other contamination incidents in the late 1950s and early 1960s contributed to gnawing doubts about the many "miracles" of the modern age. In addition to growing public wariness about the health and environmental costs of the atomic age, three other crises played a particular role in setting the stage for *Silent Spring*.

The cranberry crisis, 1959

On November 9, 1959, the US Secretary of Health, Education and Welfare shocked the nation with his recommendation that consumers refrain from purchasing cranberries (and cranberry products) from the 1957, 1958, and 1959 cranberry crops, because samples from those crops were shown to be contaminated with the weed killer, aminotriazole. Aminotriazole had been registered with the US Department of Agriculture (USDA) for nonfood use, and for use on cranberry bogs—but only for use after the berries were harvested. But in 1957, some cranberry growers in the Pacific Northwest used aminotriazole prior to harvest, and much of that year's crop from the Northwest was embargoed. By 1958, toxicity studies established that aminotriazole was carcinogenic in rodents, and a closer scrutiny of cranberry harvesting practices revealed that pre-harvest application of the weed killer was more widespread than previously thought across the United States (Lear, 2009, pp. 359–360; Janzen, 2010, pp. 87–91).

In the fall of 1959, the Department of Health, Education, and Welfare (HEW) issued a health alert about contamination of cranberries. Coming just weeks before American Thanksgiving, consumers were particularly attentive to the announcement, and cranberry sales plummeted. Follow-up testing after the HEW announcement established that only a small percentage of the nationwide crop was contaminated with aminotriazole, that no studies pointed to human carcinogenesis, and that the contamination itself was relatively minor. Nonetheless, the cat was out of the bag (Kreiger, 2005, p. 246).

This was the first national crisis that revolved around chemical contamination of food. The media was in high gear; *The New York Times* alone ran 29 stories on the cranberry crisis in just the two months of November and December 1959 (Janzen, 2010, p. 104). The cranberry scare revealed schisms in government agency regulatory positions, with the USDA fighting against the charges of contamination and arguing that concerns about toxicity were unwarranted, while the Food and Drug Administration (FDA) (housed at that time inside HEW) was arguing for strict regulations on chemical food residues. It also catalyzed a generalized public wariness about chemicals in food, as well as distrust of the government's ability to protect the public against food contamination.

Carson followed the cranberry scare closely. She attended public hearings held on the issue in mid-November 1959. Her letter the following day to a Fish and Wildlife Services biologist (and her former supervisor), Clarence Cottam, revealed some of the suspicions about vested interests that she would later develop in *Silent Spring*: "I am wondering whether you could persuade Drew Pearson [a nationally syndicated journalist] to investigate the all important subject of financial inducements behind certain pesticide programs" (cited in Lear, 2009, p. 360). Her letter to Cottam also made clear how acutely she understood the broader political implications, especially for her purposes, of the cranberry crisis: "The cranberry crisis has, I believe, been a wonderful thing in opening up the problem for a public that has been blissfully unaware that food carries anything in the way of contamination" (cited in Lear, 2009, p. 360).

Minamata disease

Minamata is a small town on the southernmost island of Japan. In the 1950s, it was both a fishing community and an industrial center. One of the largest industries in town, which rapidly expanded after World War II, was the Chisso Corporation, producing chemical fertilizers and chemicals for a wide range of industrial and medicinal purposes. The company used inorganic mercury as a chemical catalyst, producing methylmercury as a waste by-product—which it dumped directly into Minamata Bay (and continued to do so until 1968) (Jenks, 2010, p. 14).

The cats were what caught everyone's attention at first. In the early 1950s, residents noticed deaths and odd behaviors in the cats that hung out around the Minamata waterfront cadging fish scraps from the fishing fleet: convulsions, screeching, biting themselves, foaming at the mouth, flinging themselves into the ocean. But it wasn't just the cats. Dogs and birds, too, started having convulsions and exhibiting inexplicable behaviors. By the mid-1950s, many residents also suffered neurological symptoms, including tremors and convulsions, deafness, loss of speech, numbness, loss of muscle control, and, for more than 50 people, painful and protracted deaths.

Many newborns were deformed and disabled. While medical experts were initially puzzled, the residents almost immediately associated their troubles with pollution from the Chisso factory. By 1957, the medical community had caught up, and investigations confirmed that the victims—human and nonhuman alike—were suffering from mercury poisoning. The only source could be the mercury wastewater being dumped by the Chisso plant into the harbor. As most of the local population relied heavily on seafood as a mainstay of their diet, the mercury worked its way through the seafood chain, and people were being poisoned, literally, by the food they ate.

With this discovery, the wagons were circled: Chisso denied that it was the source of contamination (although there was no credible alternative source); the Japan Chemical Industry Association in 1959 produced a report claiming the disease could not possibly be linked with mercury; the Japanese Ministry of International Trade and Industry—one of the most powerful agencies within the government, whose mandate was industrial development—suspended all ongoing government scientific studies on Minamata (Jenks, 2010, p. 19). In response, thousands of outraged fishermen and their families mounted the first public environmental protest in modern Japan, storming the factory, picketing Chisso's headquarters, and petitioning politicians for action. The prefectural government imposed a partial ban on the sale of fish caught in Minamata Bay, and Chisso redirected its wastewater outflow but not its industrial practices (thus, ironically, polluting a wider area), but the protesters were widely denounced. In the words of one observer, the 1959 militancy of the fishing community was a step ahead of the more radical popular politics that would come in the following decade (Jenks, 2010, p. 19). In a bid to end the attention, Chisso management in 1959 offered the fishermen small "sympathy payments" to compensate them for "dirtying their waters"—without accepting responsibility for what, by then, had been dubbed "Minamata disease."

The controversy (but not the suffering) died down until 1965, when mercury poisoning was confirmed in another community, Niigata, further north. In Niigata, the source was another chemical company's mercury wastewater outflow into the nearby river. It wasn't until the late 1960s that the Japanese government belatedly acknowledged the official cause of Minamata disease, opening the door for compensation and liability proceedings that still continue today. By 2010, there were 2,265 "officially certified" victims of Minamata disease in Japan, 1,784 of whom had died; another 10,000 are being compensated for medical expenses for problems that are "likely to be" Minamata disease (National Institute for Minamata Disease, 2012).

The scandal of Minamata disease in Japan didn't press into the general American consciousness until the early 1970s, ignited by two striking publications: in 1969, the Japanese writer Michiko Ishimure catalyzed public outrage with her second book on Minamata disease, *Paradise in the Sea of Sorrow*; and then, in 1972, photographers Eugene and Aileen Smith published a remarkable photo essay in *Life* magazine on the victims of the disease, including what is indisputably the most iconic image from Minamata, "Tomoko Uemara in Her Bath," a photograph of a mother cradling her severely deformed naked daughter in a bath.

By the early 1970s, Minamata disease had also come home, as it were. Extensive mercury contamination of several rivers in Western Ontario, Canada, was discovered in 1970 after people in two First Nations tribes started falling ill with the same neurological syndromes as their counterparts in Japan. Doctors from Japan who were familiar with Minamata helped to diagnose the outbreak, caused, again, by an industrial company, Dryden Chemicals, dumping mercury waste into the river system. The Ontario provincial government ordered Dryden to stop dumping in 1970, and told the local communities to stop eating fish or drinking water from the English-Wabigoon river system, but by then there had been eight years of mercury contamination. In 2011, a team of Japanese doctors who returned to Ontario to conduct follow-up studies established that native peoples in the region are still experiencing health problems from the persisting contamination (Harada et al., 2011).

Knowledge of the crisis in Minamata was circulating as Carson was writing *Silent Spring* in the late 1950s, even if it was not foremost in the public conversation in the United States. In the scientific literature with which Carson would be familiar, the Minamata story was quickly rolling out.[13] Carson doesn't mention Minamata in *Silent Spring*, and it didn't provoke the same level of American public anxiety as the cranberry crisis, but Minamata added to the nagging worry about the ways in which unseen chemical contamination was a growing threat to environment and health.

Thalidomide 1957-1962

In 1954, a small German drug manufacturer developed what seemed to be a promising sedative, anti-insomnia, and anti-nausea drug: thalidomide. By 1957, the drug was widely distributed in the global market and it was eventually available in 46 countries, in most of those as an over-the-counter (not prescription) drug (Zimmer, 2010). One of the reasons for its widespread popularity was that it was found to be an effective remedy for morning sickness, and quickly became the drug of choice for pregnant women. The drug manufacturers heavily promoted this use—it seemed to promise a never-ending market.

But the dark side of this "wonder drug" was quick to emerge. By 1959, doctors in Australia and Europe, especially Germany where the drug had its widest and earliest distribution, were recording stunning numbers of children born with severely stunted and misshaped hands, and, worse, with "flipper" appendages instead of limbs. This sudden appearance of "phocomelia," a previously rare condition, was too remarkable to be ignored or to be mere chance. Medical suspicion almost immediately fell on thalidomide, but the drug manufacturer dissembled and denied any possible link to their star drug. Within two years, a German pediatrician and an Australian obstetrician established the link to thalidomide, and by 1961 there was a worldwide rush to restrict, then ban, the drug from distribution. In 1962, Canada was the last country to ban thalidomide, but not before more than 10,000 newborns with thalidomide deformities were reported worldwide.

Fewer than 20 infants in the United States were born with thalidomide deformities—almost all of them to recent immigrants from Europe, although a few to mothers who received thalidomide as pre-release doctors' samples.[14] Remarkably, thalidomide was never distributed in the United States, all thanks to the heroic efforts of one FDA investigator, Dr. Frances Kelsey. The Kelsey story is an endlessly fascinating saga of institutional politics, scientific doggedness, and an outsider's willingness to buck the system of cozy institutional relationships between manufacturers and regulators (precisely the sort of coziness that Carson spotlighted).

Thalidomide was licensed to an American drug company, Merrell, which filed an application in 1960 with the FDA to distribute the drug in the United States. The presumed easy review of a sedative with few side-effects and low toxicity was assigned to the newest FDA employee, Dr. Kelsey. Kelsey was new to the FDA but was essentially mid-career at that point, and she came to the FDA with considerable pharmacological experience. Kelsey immediately saw problems with Merrell's application—she thought the supporting test data was incomplete and unconvincing. Over the next few months, she kept returning their application for further testing and clarification. She also caught wind of some of the investigations in Europe and the rising concerns about thalidomide there. She thought Merrell's application was weak and she suspected that they were hiding some of the emerging evidence of problems with thalidomide.

In turn, Merrell executives were outraged at Kelsey; they had expected an easy pass for their drug application. They pushed back hard against what they saw as an obstinate employee, accusing her of libel and obstructionism; between September 1960 and November 1961, they contacted Kelsey's supervisors at the FDA more than 50 times to complain about Kelsey, to demand her removal, and to push vigorously for approval of thalidomide without further delay (Daemmrich, 2002, p. 154). Kelsey was able to fend them off; she held firm against enormous pressure long enough that by late 1961 the evidence against thalidomide was so strong that the application was scuttled.

Kelsey complained to her supervisors about the pressure tactics of the company and recorded the response in this 1962 memo:

> I [Kelsey] did bring up in a staff meeting the fact that I considered [FDA] Medical Officers were at times subject to excessive pressure. I was told that this was a normal hazard of the job and if I did not like it, I should seek employment elsewhere. I tried to put across the concept that in some cases, expediency might dictate that another alternative to quitting might be to yield to pressure and that therefore I felt some attention should be given to the fact that certain companies did seem to be exerting too much pressure.
> (cited in Daemmrich, 2002, pp. 154–155)

Although Kelsey didn't get as much support at the FDA as she deserved, she became a public heroine, and in 1962 President Kennedy gave her the "President's Award for Distinguished Federal Civilian Service."

Discussion of problems with thalidomide was circulating in scientific outlets in the late 1950s, but it was not much in the public domain until 1962, when it exploded into view as a full-fledged health calamity and it quickly became *the* headline story around the world. In the American public media, as Carson's *Silent Spring* was rolling out, magazines and newspapers ran shocking photographs of children with "flipper" limbs. *Life* magazine ran a list of the worldwide trade names thalidomide was marketed under, warning people to turn in those drugs immediately (Mulliken, 1962, p. 29). Kelsey's role was much heralded, with newspapers such as *The New York Times* trumpeting that "Doctor's actions bar birth defects: A woman doctor was reported today to have prevented the birth of perhaps thousands of babies with missing arms or legs" (*The New York Times*, July 16, 1962).

Thalidomide marked a sea change in public awareness about the costs of modern "miracles." Coming hard on the heels of the cranberry crisis, radiation fallout, and industrial scandals such as Minamata, the thalidomide saga was not only described as a health crisis, but as a crisis of confidence in institutions that had previously been held in high regard. *US News & World Report* ran an investigative story on "New Drugs—How Good are the Safeguards?" (August 13, 1962). The September 1, 1962 issue of the *Saturday Review* ran several hard-hitting feature stories about the crisis in credibility that the thalidomide scandal provoked: "Where is Science Taking Us?," a lengthy excerpt from the New York Academy of Sciences about the conflict of interest in drug testing and the need for a regulatory office with more clout than the current FDA; a lengthy report titled "The Unfinished Story of Thalidomide," which presented an astonishing log of the day-by-day pressures brought by the drug manufacturer on Kelsey and detailing the chummy relationships that typically prevailed between regulators and drug manufacturers; and a laudatory article about Dr. Kelsey, "The Feminine Conscience of FDA."[15]

Carson admired Kelsey, although they barely knew one another. The only time they met, as far as we know, is when Kelsey attended a meeting of the Audubon Naturalist Society in 1962, just a few days after the publication of *Silent Spring*, at which Carson made brief remarks. Kelsey apparently participated with Carson in the question-and-answer period. In another speech a few days later, Carson cited Kelsey's work to underscore the need for genetic testing of chemicals before they were released into the environment (cited in Lear, 2009, p. 423). With the thalidomide scandal breaking at the same time that *Silent Spring* was published, Carson drew a direct line between the two. A *New York Post* story in September 1962 quoted Carson as saying, "It is all of a piece, thalidomide and pesticides—they represent our willingness to rush ahead and use something new without knowing what the results are going to be" (cited in Brinkley, 2012).

* * *

Poisoned food, poisoned water, poisonous drugs, atomic fallout. In 1962, *Silent Spring* was released to a public that was growing wary of corporate malfeasance, vested interests, and vast institutions beyond their control (including government agencies) that were increasingly being shown not to be acting in the best interest of the public. As one author notes, the early 1960s was ushering in an "epoch of incredulity" (Daemmrich, 2002, p. 137). The public was ready for *Silent Spring*'s message. As compelling as *Silent Spring* was in its own terms, it became an overnight sensation because the world was rising to meet it. It was the right book, published at the right time.

For further discussion/exploration

- Tour your local hardware store and take note of how many pesticides there are, and what they are called. Do the names suggest anything about power relationships between humans and "pests"?
- For the pesticides on your list, above, see what publicly available health and safety information you can find about each one.
- List the cultural assumptions that Carson was critiquing. Do any/all of them still hold sway today? Why, or why not?
- Examine the "National Priorities List" (formerly called "Superfund") maintained by the Environmental Protection Agency (EPA)—an inventory of the most critically polluted places in the United States. How many of these are military, or ex-military, sites?

3

Needless Havoc: Carson's Case Against Pesticides

The ideology that pesticides were the means to the end goal of controlling nature—against which Carson was writing—was eloquently laid bare by the 1943–1947 Department of Agriculture's Yearbook, subtitled "Science in Farming." In eerily militarized Baconian terms, one of the authors exults:

> Since creation, men have joined to conquer nature or separated to fight for her fruits. Science has furnished them increasingly effective tools to make nature more productive and increasingly effective weapons for seizing a larger share of the goods produced.
> When men, as allies, use science to get the most from each acre, each worker, each machine, each animal, they make it possible for the earth or a part of it to support more people . . . For example, 140 million Americans now live in relative peacefulness in an area where a fraction of a million Indians once fought for hunting grounds. Scientific progress enables some people to live better, and more people to live.
> (Johnson, 1947, p. 920)

As I have argued thus far, *Silent Spring* can very much be read as a manifesto by Carson against exactly this ideological context—the boosterist embrace of militarized, "miracle of science" definitions of "progress," in which nature is reduced to spoils of war. One historian defines the pre-*Silent Spring* era as one in which Americans "assumed science was good, that chemicals were necessary, that their use would be governed by experts, that these experts could be trusted, and that the side-effects of chemical use would be negligible" (Dunlap, 1981, p. 235).

Carson understood that while pesticides were *products* of this ideology, they also acted to advance its goals. In post-war/Cold War America, pesticides had the lead role in the drama of "man against nature," and it was into this fray that Carson stepped.[1]

Carson did not undertake original research about pesticides. *Silent Spring* is, instead, a synthesis of scientific research conducted by others—much of it, in its original form, often abstruse and highly technical. One of Carson's greatest contributions was her ability to "translate" the scientific literature for public consumption. As a scientist and a former insider at the US Fish and Wildlife Service, Carson was aware of and privy to many of the reports on pesticides that circulated only inside government agencies or that only other government scientists cared about. She was also a keen collector of public information, including the work of several activists and community groups raising concerns about pesticides, which she then wove together with the scientific information into a coherent whole.

Carson was not the first to point to evidence of the dangers of pesticides. By the time she started writing *Silent Spring* in the late 1950s, the scientific literature on pesticide hazards, including documentation of several massive fish kills and uncovering the knowledge that DDT would pass through to infants from mothers' milk, was piling up. Indeed, it was this literature that Carson pulled together. And that was one of her great contributions: before Carson, published studies about pesticide dangers were scattered throughout various specialized scientific outlets, and the evidence was spotty and in some cases contradictory or uncertain. Carson brought coherence to the field. Like assembling a jigsaw puzzle (key pieces of which were stashed away in agency file cabinets), she pulled together the pieces in a way that made a discernable picture. This was not easy and there were many contradictions. For example, she observed to a friend that individual doctors might document physical

NEEDLESS HAVOC

illnesses related to pesticides, but the American Medical Association and the Public Health Service were evasive in taking a stand (cited in Hynes, 1989, p. 33).

For Carson, *Silent Spring* was the culmination of two decades of mounting concern about the use of pesticides—her own concern, and that of many inside scientific circles. Linda Lear details Carson's path towards *Silent Spring*, dating her concern to the earliest years of her professional career:

> Carson's concern about poisons and pollution can be documented as early as 1938 and probably began even earlier. She was personally and professionally opposed to Fish and Wildlife Service predator control policies throughout her federal career not simply because they were based on killing certain animals, but because they ignored the ecology of the total habitat. While writing the FWS "Conservation Bulletins" on fish and fisheries during the war, she read the reports of Cottam and Higgins on DDT residues present in inland and marine fish and like her mentors, worried about increased contamination.
>
> (Lear, 1993, p. 30)

But it was three specific events in the late 1950s that propelled her towards *Silent Spring*. All three involved disastrous consequences from indiscriminate aerial spraying of pesticides. Lear continues:

> The first involved the controversial campaign undertaken by USDA in 1957 to eradicate the imported fire ant from the southern states by massive applications of dieldrin and heptachlor, two of the most persistent and most toxic new pesticides. Reports of wildlife damage brought a chorus of criticism from conservation groups. Carson read these reports, discussed them with her friends, attended USDA briefings as an Audubon member, and followed the acrimonious pesticide debate within the National Academy of Science/National Research Council on which her friend and former supervisor Clarence Cottam served.
>
> About the same time she also received information on bird mortality caused by the aerial spraying of DDT mixed in fuel oil for mosquito control in the coastal counties of northern

Massachusetts. Friend and fellow writer Olga Owens Huckins' home and bird sanctuary in Duxbury had been subjected to that spraying. Saddened and angry over the numbers of birds that had perished, Huckins wrote to the *Boston Herald* in protest. She sent Carson a copy of the published letter in January 1958 urging her to find someone in Washington to help stop the spraying. In the course of sleuthing on Huckins's behalf Carson uncovered the enormity of the pesticide problem. She understood immediately that there was material for an article at least and perhaps for a book.

Finally, Carson's initial inquiries about aerial spraying took place not only during the height of the fire ant controversy, but also at a time when newspapers were full of accounts of a trial in Long Island involving shocking misuse of pesticides. Robert Cushman Murphy, noted ornithologist, director of the American Museum of Natural History, and one of Carson's early benefactors, pursued the novel strategy of attempting to enjoin the federal government from further aerial pesticide spraying. Testimony presented during the trial documented enormous damage that pesticides had done to fish, birds, wildlife, dairy cattle, gardens, livestock, and perhaps to children. The suit, which was eventually dismissed on technicalities after appeal to the Supreme Court, gathered testimony from a variety of experts. It provided Rachel Carson with "mountains of material," important collaborators such as Mary Richards and Marjorie Spock, and a wealth of expert contacts in medical and agricultural fields previously unknown to her.

(Lear, 1993, pp. 30–31)

So, what *was* Carson worried about? To the chagrin of many contemporary environmentalists, Carson is not entirely opposed to the use of pesticides. She concedes their importance to human health and agriculture, and she agrees that they have a role to play in modern food systems. What she *is* opposed to is:

- pesticide use that is unjustified, or justified on the flimsiest evidence, without careful balancing of the severity of the alleged pest problem against the problems caused by pesticides;

- the tendency for an "automatic" recourse to pesticides, for virtually every occasion—the "habit of killing" as she called it;
- pesticides applied through aerial spraying—the least controlled and most inexact way of applying pesticides, a method that maximizes the "collateral damage" deaths of all living entities in the spray path, not only the designated "pest."

Carson was also deeply worried about the pace of development of new chemicals; a speed with which an already-inadequate regulatory system could not keep up. She further was convinced that evidence of insect resistance to pesticides and "rebounds" in insect populations was widely witnessed but widely ignored. And she was alarmed by the health consequences of pesticide exposure, consequences that she felt were only barely known or accommodated. So, it was both the nature of the new chemicals themselves Carson was concerned about, as well as humans' reckless use of them.

Carson offered possibly the most concise explication of her core arguments—a kind of condensed *Silent Spring*—in a January 1963 speech to the Garden Club of America:

> This is a time when forces of a very different nature often prevail—forces careless of life or deliberately destructive of it and of the essential web of living relationships.
>
> My particular concern, as you know, is with the reckless use of chemicals so unselective in their action that they should more appropriately be called biocides rather than pesticides . . . We should be very clear about what our cause is. What do we oppose? What do we stand for? If you read some of my industry-oriented reviewers you would think that I am opposed to any efforts to control insects or other organisms. This of course is not my position . . .
>
> It is my conviction that if we automatically call in the spray planes or reach for the aerosol bomb when we have an insect problem we are resorting to crude methods of a rather low scientific order . . .
>
> I criticize the present heavy reliance upon biocides on several grounds: First, on the grounds of their inefficiency . . . also because

as now used they promote resistance among insects ... and often provoke resurgences of the very insect they seek to control, because they have killed off its natural controls. Or they cause some other organism suddenly to rise to nuisance status.

(Carson, 1998b, pp. 212–214)

Carson finds the world of pesticides to be a weirdly distorted realm, surpassing, she would say in *Silent Spring*, the "imaginings of the brothers Grimm" (p. 39). This is a world where forests and plants have become reservoirs of poison, where bees produce poisonous honey from contaminated pollen, where insects die from plants they haven't even touched. This is the dystopia produced by the profligate development and reckless use of compounds, the consequences of which humans know pitifully little.

The elixirs of death

Although Carson is most closely associated with her analysis of the dangers of DDT, in fact she compiled persuasive evidence of the environmental and health havoc wrought by more than a dozen insecticides and herbicides that she specifically names, among them: the *chlorinated hydrocarbons* (such as DDT, chlordane, dieldrin, aldrin, endrin); the *organic phosphorous* insecticides (including parathion, malathion, and pentachloriphenol); and several herbicides, first and foremost, 2,4-D. She was concerned about all of the synthetic chemicals pouring out of American factories—chemicals that, in her estimation, "differ[ed] sharply from the simpler insecticides of prewar days" (p. 25) in their biological potency and imprudent use. DDT came under Carson's special scrutiny.

DDT: The "gateway drug"

DDT was the darling of post-war America. In a 1945 US War Department propaganda film, this "miraculous white powder" was credited with saving thousands of lives—in the European theater of war where it protected civilians and soldiers against typhus, cholera, and lice, and in the Pacific where tons of DDT were dumped on battleground atolls across the Pacific, saving Allied soldiers from the scourge of malaria and dengue fever.[2] The war proved the efficacy of aerial spraying of insecticides, and, as the War Department (later to become the Defense Department) promised, as soon as the war was over this miracle would be brought home. The sonorous voice-over in the film narrates the promise:

> In the Pacific, DDT goes to war against malaria in a big way—by airplane. On D-Day at Morotai, we hit both enemies at the same time. The Jap (*sic.*) and disease. Simultaneous with the bombing of our two-legged enemy, we went after the mosquito with DDT spray, and as a result of the spray malaria was already under control before our troops set foot on the island. The Japanese did not live long enough to enjoy the island rid of mosquitoes by DDT.
> Yes, today DDT is necessarily a military weapon. We're turning it out by the thousands of tons, but every ounce is needed for the war effort. When the fascist is finally beaten though, DDT will be available to all.
> Already it has been found to be highly effective against many kinds of agricultural insect pests. It will aid in stamping out disease around the world. And the homecoming of the healthiest army in military history will be in no small part due to DDT, our great new weapon for war today and peace tomorrow.

As soon as the War Department released its monopoly on the use of DDT, the blitz to get it into the domestic market began. With its wartime halo, DDT was heavily promoted as the insecticide of choice—for agriculture, for the homeowner, for the gardener, for the housewife. The Department of Agriculture was a major cheerleader for DDT: in its 1952 *Yearbook of Agriculture*, the agency hailed DDT as "one of our safest all-around insecticides" based on its "cost, ease of handling, safety to humans, effectiveness in destroying the pest, and safety to wildlife."[3] DDT was manufactured by several companies, including Ciba, Montrose, Pennwalt, and Velsicol, and became one of the most widely used chemicals in the United States. Between 1945, when it was released for public use, and 1972, when it was banned, an estimated 1.3 billion pounds of DDT was used in the United States (USEPA, 1975).

In 1959, as Carson was writing *Silent Spring*, DDT use in the United States was at what would be its all-time peak, an estimated 80 million pounds in that year alone (USEPA, 1975). Carson's review of the scientific literature on DDT and her correspondence with many scientists inside and outside various government agencies, alarmed her. As the first mass-produced synthetic pesticide, Carson saw DDT as the stalking horse for even more powerful pesticides, the first step on to the pesticide treadmill. Since DDT was released for civilian use, she said we trapped ourselves in a cycle of escalation in which ever more toxic materials must be found. Insects, "in a triumphant vindication of Darwin's principle of the survival of the fittest" (p. 18), rapidly develop resistance to insecticides—thus, different and more powerful insecticides need to be applied, to which those insects will develop resistance. Carson also points to "flareback" (p. 18) a well-documented resurgence of insects following spraying—to which, again, even more spraying seems the only resort.

Carson lays out the basic structure and biological uptake processes of DDT in her chapter, "Elixirs of Death." In addition to being the "gateway drug," DDT had specific characteristics that made it, in Carson's view, the first "biocide."

Fatty tissue storage and generational pass-through

In mammals, DDT is stored in the fat (especially the liver, kidneys, and intestines), and once in the body it is "biomagnified" so that even a small uptake of DDT will produce a net result of considerable DDT body burden. Carson explains that fatty tissue storage of DDT begins with even the smallest intake of the chemical. The fatty tissue deposits then act as biological magnifiers that can produce an increase of 100 times or more of DDT concentrations in the body. Because pesticides are very slowly excreted, chronic and persistent storage in the body can cause degenerative changes to the liver in the first instance, and to other organs in sequence.

Moreover, the experimental literature told Carson that chlorinated hydrocarbons such as DDT could easily pass through the placenta barrier, passing the poison from mother to child.

Ecosystem bioaccumulation and magnification

Carson prefigured public awareness of "bioaccumulation"—a process whereby toxic substances are absorbed faster than they are lost—and "biomagnification"—whereby a substance increases in concentration as it moves up the food chain. In Carson's view, both bioaccumulation and biomagnification underscored the dangers of exposure to radioactive materials as well as to pesticides. She first raised this concern in the Preface she wrote for the 1961 edition of the reissued *The Sea Around Us*, talking about radiation:

> What happens then to the careful calculation of a "maximum permissible level" [of radioactivity]? For the tiny organisms are eaten by larger ones and so on up the food chain to man. By such a process, tuna over an area of a million square miles surrounding the Bikini bomb test developed a degree of radioactivity enormously higher than that of the sea water.
>
> (1961, p. xii)

Turning this understanding to her investigation of pesticides, Carson writes about the "sinister" (p. 30) way that DDT and related chemicals were passed along from one organism to the next all the way up the food chain. If a field of grain is sprayed with DDT, she informs readers, and the grain then fed to hens, the hens will lay eggs containing DDT. If a field of hay is sprayed, and the hay then fed to cows, their milk will contain DDT; further, Carson points out, if butter is made from that milk, it will contain DDT at a concentration of approximately 20 times that of the milk. Small exposures to DDT, Carson informed shocked readers, would "biomagnify" up the food chain and through various types of foodstuffs—fatty foodstuffs, the most of all.

Carson returns throughout *Silent Spring* to the threat of poisonings conveyed up the food chain: birds or higher-order animals didn't need to be exposed directly to poisons to die from them. Carson tells several stories that demonstrate the effect of bioaccumulation and magnification, few as startling as the story of the massive die-off of grebes (a freshwater diving bird) in Clear Lake in California in the mid-1950s following a program of spraying of DDD, a compound related to DDT, to kill gnats.

Carson tells how grebes started to die off following the first spraying for gnats in 1954. But by the third spraying in 1957, the number of grebes found dead and dying was extraordinary. Bird pathologists could find no evidence of infectious disease or other usual cause of death. One researcher finally decided to look in the fatty tissues for evidence of contamination—finding DDD at an extraordinary concentration of 1,600 parts per million. But this was even more puzzling than the unanticipated bird deaths themselves—the maximum concentration of DDD sprayed on and around the lake was one-fiftieth part per million. Carson asks the question that is surely on the readers' minds of how such high levels of DDD could be found in the grebes. The answer lies in the food chain: the birds accumulated poison from the fish they ate, which picked up the poison from the small organisms *they* ate. Plankton in Clear Lake was found to contain about 5 parts per million of the insecticide—about 25 times the maximum concentration that was ever found in the water itself. Plankton-eating fish were found to have 40 to 300 parts per million. Carnivorous fish (such as the brown bullhead in Clear Lake) that eat other fish, midges, worms, and crayfish showed even more astounding concentrations—one particular fish analyzed had 2,500 parts per million. "It was a house-that-Jack-built sequence, in which the large carnivores had eaten the smaller carnivores, that had eaten the herbivores, that had eaten the plankton, that had absorbed the poison from the water" (p. 52).

Carson continues to narrate the catastrophe. A short time after the last spraying of the lake, there was no chemical trace of DDD found in the water. It seemed to have dispersed as quickly as the sprayers had predicted it would. But, shockingly, Carson says, the poison had not really left the lake; it had merely "gone into the fabric of the life of the lake" (p. 52). Two years after the last DDD spraying, investigators found that the plankton still contained more than 5 parts per million. Most plankton has a short lifespan; several "generations" of plankton had bloomed and died in the intervening two years. But the poison—even having been apparently cleansed from the water itself—kept passing from one plankton generation to the next.

The poison did not have a tight grip only on the plankton. The plankton was merely the "original concentrator," the base of the food chain. A year after the last spraying of DDD, all the birds, frogs, and fish were found to have DDD in their bodies—even fish that had hatched nine months after the last spraying of DDD. Some of the birds, long after the last spraying, had built up DDD concentrations of more than 2,000 parts per million. Carson tells the sad denouement: the nesting colonies of the grebes dwindled—from more than 1,000 pairs before the first insecticide treatment, to about 30 pairs in 1960. Carson reported on the scientific evidence, then emerging, that DDT was implicated in the reproductive failures among top-of-the-food-chain raptors such as ospreys, falcons, and eagles. In some parts of the United States, reported declines in eagle populations were putting the bird at near-extinction levels. The mechanism of DDT's effect on reproduction in raptors was not known as Carson was writing *Silent Spring*, but energetic pursuit of the mystery of the disappearing raptors, inspired in part by Carson's work, continued throughout the 1960s,. By the late 1960s, the evidence was widely accepted that DDT blocked the absorption of calcium in adult birds and caused thin-shelled eggs that could not protect bird embryos through hatching. Evidence of the sharp decline in raptor populations associated with DDT was instrumental in its 1972 ban.[4]

Persistence and build-up

Researchers working on DDT knew that it was a persistent chemical, even though they didn't know then, as we do now, that its half-life (the time it takes for half the compound to degrade) in soils is 2–15 years, and in aquatic environments it is 150 years (National Pesticide Information Center, 1999). Carson startled her readership with facts about the persistence of chemicals in the environment; a persistence measured in years, not merely in weeks or months. Aldrin, for example, she told her readers, could easily be found four years after its application. Toxaphene, once applied to soils, persists enough that it can still kill termites ten years later. Benzene hexachloride, ten years; heptachlor, at least nine; chlordane, more than 12 years. These findings would have shocked her dawn-of-the-pesticide-age readers.

Carson laid out the evidence that the persistence of the chlorinated hydrocarbons such as DDT meant that seemingly moderate applications of insecticides over a period of years could build up astonishing quantities in soil. The alleged "harmlessness" of an application of DDT meant little if it was repeatedly applied to cropland. Potato soils, she says, have been found to contain up to 15 pounds of DDT per acre; cornfield soils have been found with 19 pounds per acre. One cranberry bog contained 34 pounds per acre. DDT in apple orchards accumulated at a rate that was almost equivalent to the rate of its application.

DDT today

- The first country to ban DDT was Hungary, in 1968, followed by Norway and Sweden in 1970; banned from use in the United States in 1972, in the UK in 1984; the major reasons for DDT's prohibition were because it persists in the environment, it accumulates in fatty tissues of humans and other animals, it is highly toxic and was demonstrated to be especially dangerous to reproduction in raptors and fish-eating birds, and it was becoming ineffective due to growing insect resistance.

- The 2004 Stockholm Convention on Persistent Organic Pollutants (POPs) banned its use worldwide (for countries that signed the Convention), with exceptions made for its continued use in anti-malaria insect-control programs; the US government is not a party to the Stockholm Convention.

- As of 2008, DDT was still manufactured in India, China, and North Korea, with India being by far the largest user; several countries are contemplating re-introducing DDT for malaria control (Van den Berg, 2008).

- DDT residues are still found throughout the United States, both in people's bodies and in ecosystems, and given its half-life, this will be the case for several more decades.

Chlordane and heptachlor

Velsicol was the chemical company most vociferous in its threats of legal action against *Silent Spring*'s publisher in the lead-up to the book's release. At the time *Silent Spring* was published, Velsicol was the sole US manufacturer of chlordane—an insecticide and herbicide that had been particularly successfully marketed for household use on lawns, for termite control, for wood treatment, and as an indoor insecticide spray.

In Carson's view, chlordane (another chlorinated hydrocarbon), was even worse than DDT—carrying the most nasty characteristics of DDT, plus a few of its own. Chlordane, like DDT, had long persistence in soil, on food, and on other surfaces. Moreover, "Chlordane makes use of all available portals to enter the body. It may be absorbed through the skin, may be breathed in as a spray or dust, and of course is absorbed from the digestive tract if residues are swallowed. Like all other chlorinated hydrocarbons, its deposits build up in the body in cumulative fashion" (p. 31). Carson quotes a pharmacologist, Dr. Lehman, who described chlordane in 1950 as one of the most toxic of insecticides and who warned that anyone handling it could be poisoned.

Heptachlor (a constituent of chlordane) was marketed as a separate product, and it was found to be even *more* toxic than chlordane, though slightly less toxic to fish than DDT (though still disastrously poisonous). One of the peculiarities of heptachlor is that in animal tissues it assumes a new, more toxic form known as "heptachlor epoxide". Throughout *Silent Spring*, Carson details chlordane deaths and poisonings of pesticide workers and end-user consumers. She also implicates chlordane use in large-scale poisonings of ecosystems, including the fire ant fiasco, described below.

Chlordane and heptachlor today[5]

- Chlordane was used in the United States from 1948 to 1978 as a pesticide on agricultural crops, lawns, and gardens, and as a fumigating agent. In 1978, EPA canceled the use of chlordane on food crops and phased out other above-ground uses over the next five years. From 1983 to 1988, chlordane's only approved use was to control subterranean termites. It is highly toxic to "non-target" animals such as birds, bees, aquatic organisms (including fish), and earthworms.

- In 1988, *all* approved uses of chlordane in the United States were terminated. In 1997, the world's last producer of chlordane, Velsicol, announced it would phase out production; but as of 2011, its status is unclear and there appear to still be US exports of chlordane overseas.

- Like the other chlorinated hydrocarbons, chlordane is highly persistent and bioaccumulative; it has been found in soils decades after the last application. In 2012, autopsies conducted on dead birds in New Jersey found chlordane residues in the birds; investigations lead researchers to examine insects and grubs emerging from golf courses and other turf areas that had decades earlier seen heavy chlordane use. The insects had high chlordane concentrations.

- Chlordane is rated by the EPA as a "probable" human carcinogen, with the potential to cause central nervous system effects. Since it highly accumulates in fatty tissue, its link to breast cancer has long been suspected, but not proven.

- Chlordane is among the "dirty dozen" POPs identified and banned worldwide by the 2004 Stockholm Convention.

- Most uses of heptachlor—to kill termites in homes, insects on crops, and for wood treatment—were ended in 1978; it was fully banned in 1988 in the United States.

- Heptachlor is one of the "dirty dozen" POPs identified and banned worldwide by the 2004 Stockholm Convention.

- Heptachlor is classified as a "probable" human carcinogen.

- It is believed to be responsible for the decline of several wild bird populations, including kestrels in the Columbia River basin.

- In 2006, the Natural Resources Defense Council reported that heptachlor was still widely used in many developing countries.

- Researchers in Japan, the United States, Turkey, Argentina, and Egypt have all recently reported finding heptachlor-contaminated soil in farming districts.

Aldrin, dieldrin, endrin

Carson identifies these three chemically-related chlorinated hydrocarbon insecticides as among the "most violently poisonous," causing an "appalling destruction of wildlife" (p. 34). Aldrin and dieldrin (the latter named for a German chemist, Diels), were introduced to the American market in the late 1940s, primarily as controls for soil insects and for direct application on certain crops, especially corn and potatoes and fruit. Carson reports on research that showed dieldrin was about five times as toxic as DDT when swallowed, but 40 times as toxic when absorbed through the skin in solution. Tested on birds such as quail and pheasants, it was 40–50 times as toxic as DDT. As with other chlorinated hydrocarbons, dieldrin concentrates in fatty tissues of mammals, causes severe damage to the liver, and disrupts the central nervous system.

Despite this baseline information about these three insecticides, Carson makes the point that there are vast gaps in knowledge about the long-term impacts of these chemicals. Chemists, Carson said, were able to outpace medical and scientific knowledge— able to create new chemicals at such a pace that monitoring analysis could not keep up. As Carson was writing, there was virtually no medical literature that examined how dieldrin is stored, excreted, or distributed in the human body. However, there was preliminary research that established that dieldrin could be stored for years in human and other animal fatty tissues, and would be activated, diabolically, in times of stress when fat reserves were called upon.

The richest source of evidence of dieldrin's effect in the human body came, Carson said, from antimalarial campaigns run by the World Health Organization (WHO) in the late 1950s. In many parts of the world, the WHO had replaced DDT with dieldrin, because the mosquitoes were becoming resistant to DDT.[6] Carson tells the impact this had on the front-line pesticide workers—those with the greatest exposure to dieldrin. As soon as dieldrin was substituted for DDT, Carson says, "cases of poisoning among the spraymen began to occur. The seizures were severe—from half to all (varying in the different programs) of the men affected went into convulsions and several died. Some had convulsions as long as four months after the last exposure" (p. 33).

Aldrin is a "mysterious" substance closely chemically related to dieldrin, Carson reports, but even more toxic than dieldrin when directly applied to plants and insects. (Sunlight and bacteria change aldrin into dieldrin, so we mostly find dieldrin in the environment.) In aldrin, Carson sees the "menacing shadow of the future" (p. 34) in its proven effects on damaging animal reproduction. She is alarmed to report that there was, at that time, no evidence as to whether the same effect will turn up in human beings, but, to underscore one of her central points, she reminds the reader that despite lack of knowledge of the effects of this chemical on human health, it is routinely sprayed on agricultural lands. Subsequent investigation has established that both aldrin and dieldrin are "estrogenic" chemicals, about which I provide more information in Chapter 4.

The *most* toxic of this hydrocarbon group of pesticides, Carson says, is endrin: "a little twist in its molecular structure makes it 5 times as poisonous [as aldrin]. It makes the progenitor of all this group of insecticides, DDT, seem by comparison almost harmless. It is 15 times as poisonous as DDT to mammals, 30 times as poisonous to fish, and about 300 times as poisonous to some birds" (p. 34).

Dieldrin, aldrin, and endrin today[7]

- All three are listed on the Stockholm Convention's initial list of "dirty dozen" POPs and banned in countries that signed that Convention. Dieldrin shows particularly strong persistence, and, like most of its chemical cognates, biomagnifies.

- All uses of aldrin and dieldrin were banned in the United States in 1985 except for subsurface termite control, dipping of nonfood roots and tops, and moth-proofing in a closed manufacturing process. The EPA reports that dieldrin is still found in the environment from past uses. Both aldrin and dieldrin are readily volatized from soil sediments, and are transported by air currents; both have been found in tissues of Arctic animals thousands of miles from sites of direct application. According to the "Toxic

Substances and Disease Registry," dieldrin is almost ubiquitous in the American environment.

- Production of endrin in 1980 was reported to be a comparatively slight 100,000 pounds. Endrin's main use was as an insect, bird, and rat killer; it was also used on agricultural crops, cotton seeds, control of birds on buildings, and mice in orchards. The EPA presently considers endrin use canceled; it has not been sold or produced for general use in the United States since 1986. Its use is now banned in all of the European Union, and is banned in those countries signing the Stockholm Convention. Endrin is persistent—in soils up to 14 years—but it is broken down by sunlight.

By this point in *Silent Spring*, the casual reader is swimming in details. In part, this is because Carson genuinely wants to educate her general readership; but, in larger part, her carefulness to provide scientific and technical information is because Carson has at least two constituencies for whom she is writing. Carson has the difficult task of making sure she provides sufficient scientific evidence about the pesticides she is critiquing to establish her credibility with other scientists (and industry leaders whom she knows will attack her), while at the same time she has to make her book readable and interesting to a lay audience accustomed to reading "life of the sea" books from her. The way she does this is to tell real-world stories about the havoc wrought by these pesticides. And as she does so, she introduces her readership to the (then-new) notion of "ecosystems."

Thinking like an ecosystem

The notion of "ecosystem" would have been new to most of Carson's readers. The concept was fashioned in the 1930s by scientists such as Arthur Tansley and Charles Elton in the UK, emerging in the United States in the 1950s through scientists such as Eugene Odum. When Carson was writing, ecosystem analysis was still a young and emerging field. Carson was in direct touch with the foremost ecosystem thinkers. She was deeply influenced by British ecologist Charles Elton who, in his 1958 book, *The Ecology of Invasions of Animals and Plants,* condemned the widespread use of synthetic pesticides, declaring that "this astonishing rain of death upon so much of the earth's surface" was largely unnecessary and threatened life on the planet. Carson used this "rain of death" phrase in a letter she wrote to *The New York Times* in 1959 (cited in Foster and Clark, 2008), and it serves as the trope for her *Silent Spring* chapter, "Indiscriminately From the Skies."

Carson was even more deeply influenced by Elton's associate, Robert Rudd, a scientist in California who was studying pesticides with whom she became friends. Rudd published two articles for *The Nation* in 1959, "The Irresponsible Poisoners," and "Pesticides: The *Real* Peril." Rudd, a sophisticated leftist thinker, argued that the overuse of pesticides such as DDT was based on a misplaced prioritization of "production" over other values. He wrote, "Overproduction has settled on us like a plague . . . Chemical use to increase production is continually stressed and few stop to inquire 'why?'" (cited in Foster and Clark, 2008).

There are many echoes of Rudd's work throughout *Silent Spring,* including, specifically, Carson's argument against "productionist" values. She rhetorically asks what purpose the high-risk embrace of chemicals serves. She suggests that future historians would be aghast and amazed by our skewed values:

> How could intelligent beings seek to control a few unwanted species by a method that contaminated the entire environment and brought the threat of disease and death even to their own kind? Yet this is precisely what we have done. We have done it, moreover, for reasons that collapse the moment we examine them. We are told that the enormous and expanding use of pesticides is necessary to maintain farm production. Yet is our real problem not one of *overproduction*? [emphasis added] Our farms . . . have yielded such a staggering excess of crops that the American taxpayer in 1962 is paying out more than one billion dollars a year as the total carrying cost of the surplus-food storage program.
>
> (p. 19)

Being influenced by Rudd, but not as comfortable with espousing an explicitly radical political economy analysis, Carson follows this extraordinary passage with a quick reassurance to her readers:

> All this is not to say there is no insect problem and no need of control. I am saying, rather, that control must be geared to realities, not to mythical situations, and that the methods employed must be such that they do not destroy us along with the insects.
>
> (p. 19)

But, overall, despite her efforts to make her analysis more palatable to a wide readership, it is clear that she shares Rudd's view that the problem of pesticides is one of "values," and that the privileging of productionism and profit-seeking—regardless of collateral damage—is the root of the problem. It is worth revisiting, in this context, her astonishing diatribe against the ascendancy of the assumption that "the social good" could be defined by industry – industry that then feeds the public those "little tranquilizing pills of half truth" (p. 23). Carson's real anger usually is tamped down, but throughout *Silent Spring* she allows herself a few such moments such as this in which she unblinkingly "speaks truth to power."

For Carson, ecosystem thinking in itself and by itself represents a radical challenge to the notion of human domination over nature. In this planet's ecosystem, she is alerting her readers, humans are simply *part* of nature, and subject to the same forces of disruption. If humans disrupt nature, they cannot escape the consequences—humans are not separate from nature, somehow able to avoid the consequences of their acts. She dismisses critics who suggest that the "balance of nature" is somehow a feature of a more primitive era:

> The balance of nature is not the same today as in Pleistocene times, but it is still there: a complex, precise, and highly integrated system of relationships between living things which cannot safely be ignored any more than the law of gravity can be defied with impunity by a man perched on the edge of a cliff.
>
> (p. 218)

The term "ecology" would have been more familiar than "ecosystem" to Carson's readers, and it was through this notion of "an ecology," a natural community, that Carson introduces her readers to the idea of thinking about the interrelatedness of life. Whenever Carson introduces a new concept, she tries to make it tangible by giving it a face. So, rather than just saying "in nature, everything is connected," she draws a more evocative picture, urging readers to understand that humans are "no more removed from nature as is the robin in Michigan or the salmon in the Miramichi" (p. 169). The chain of interconnectedness is crucial to her message about how poisoning works: humans generally don't directly spray robins, but robins die nonetheless because they eat the insects, the leaves, the worms that *are* poisoned. Such interconnections, the essence of "ecology," she poignantly says, are everywhere visible and observable in the world around us.

Rather than lecture about ecology and ecosystems, Carson tells the stories of where and how it had all gone wrong. Examining two of these lengthy narratives reveals Carson's pedagogical approach.

1. Eradication of the sagebrush lands of the west

In the chapter on "Earth's Green Mantle," Carson tells the story of the sagebrush eradication program conducted throughout the west. Responding to pressures from cattle farmers, the US Forest Service started spraying thousands of pounds of herbicides throughout sagebrush lands to make way for grassland grazing for cattle. With devastating results.

Carson starts with a lyrical description of the unique sagebrush ecology. In the harsh climate of the high western plains, with dry summers and frigid winters, sagebrush emerged as the most successful plant colonizer. The sage, which grows low to the ground, can hold its purchase on steep slopes and in high winds. As a xerophyte, it can withstand long periods of drought. Over the long evolution of the plains sagebrush ecology, sage plants became the basis for the survival and success of associated animals: antelope, lizards, the sage grouse. For antelope, especially, the hardy evergreen sage provides sustenance during the long winters when most other food sources become unavailable.

Into this delicately balanced ecology comes the pesticide sprayer. Much as she set up the fabled town in her opening chapter, having set the stage of the beautiful sagebrush landscape of nature in harmony, Carson then introduces the force of evil: the land management agencies who, responding to demands from cattle farmers, set about to replace the sagebrush (which their cattle didn't eat) with grazing lands—via the means of aerial spraying the sagelands with herbicides. Carson notes that, in addition to the cattle interests, there were several industrial interests that had a stake in creating more grasslands, including grass seed producers and grass cultivation machine makers. Carson underscores the futility of this effort to establish grasslands in the high plains sagelands, since it already seemed clear that grassland couldn't thrive in such an arid climate. But, ignoring that reality, the program of sage eradication marched steadily forward. Carson narrates the inevitable destruction to the entire closely knit fabric of life:

> The antelope and the grouse will disappear along with the sage. The deer will suffer, too, and the land will be poorer for the destruction of the wild things that belong to it. Even the livestock which are the intended beneficiaries will suffer; no amount of lush green grass in summer can help the sheep starving in the winter storms for lack of the sage and bitterbrush and other wild vegetation of the plains.
>
> (p. 67)

Because of the shotgun effect of indiscriminate spraying, "nontarget" plants and animals were destroyed. Narrating the specific story of one sagebrush eradication program in the Bridger National Forest in Wyoming, "an appalling example of ecological destruction wrought by the United States Forest Service" (p. 67), Carson tells the excruciating story of the cascade of loss when more than 10,000 acres of sagelands were sprayed by the Forest Service, acting at the behest of cattle ranchers who wanted to expand their grasslands:

> The sage was killed, as intended. But so was the green, life-giving ribbon of willows that traced its way across these plains, following the meandering streams. Moose had lived in these willow thickets . . . Beaver had lived there, too, feeding on the willows, felling

them and making a strong dam across the tiny stream. Through the labor of the beavers, a lake backed up. Trout thrived . . . Waterfowl were attracted to the lake, also . . . But with the "improvement" instituted by the Forest Service, the willows went the way of the sagebrush, killed by the same impartial spray . . . What would become of the moose? Of the beavers and the little world they had constructed? A year later the answers [were evident] in the devastated landscape. The moose were gone and so were the beaver. Their principal dam had gone out for want of attention by its skilled architects, and the lake had drained away. None of the large trout were left. None could live in the tiny creek that remained, threading its way through a bare, hot land where no shade remained. The living world was shattered.

(pp. 67–68)

2. The poisoning of Sheldon, Illinois

Carson's description of yet another governmental program of eradication, this time by the Department of Agriculture in Illinois, allowed her to expand on her plaint about human carelessness for life:

> Under the philosophy that now seems to guide our destinies, nothing must get in the way of the man with the spray-gun. The incidental victims of his crusade against insects count as nothing; if robins, pheasants, raccoons, cats, or even livestock happen to inhabit the same bit of earth as the target insects and to be hit by the rain of insect-killing poisons, no one must protest.
>
> (p. 83)

In Sheldon, Illinois, in the mid-1950s, the federal and state Departments of Agriculture combined forces in an effort to stop the advance of the Japanese beetle. In 1954, the first year of aerial spraying, dieldrin was applied to 1,400 acres in Sheldon. Almost double that acreage was sprayed the following year. Spraying continued for several years, and at one point the even more toxic (but cheaper) aldrin was substituted for the original dieldrin. By 1961, more than 130,000 acres were under aerial assault. The density of insecticide was extraordinary: dieldrin was applied at a rate of about 3 pounds per acre, the equivalent of DDT applications of 150 pounds per acre.

Right from the beginning, Carson says, it was clear that heavy losses were occurring in both wildlife and domesticated animals. Some of the deaths were due to animals being in the direct path of the largely indiscriminate spraying. Some were due to what we now call "pesticide drift"—for example, many farmers reported that sheep were poisoned when they were put out to graze in a field that itself was unsprayed, but that was adjacent to a sprayed field. Many animals and birds were killed because poison came to them through the food chain. The death chain started with poisoned insects crawling out of the soil and, in many instances, lying on the surface for several days—where they were especially attractive to birds looking for an easy meal:

> The effect on the bird populations could easily have been foretold. Brown thrashers, starlings, meadowlarks, grackles, and pheasants were virtually wiped out. Robins were "almost annihilated," according to the biologists' report . . . Birds seen drinking and bathing in puddles left by rain a few days after the spraying were inevitably doomed . . . Among the mammals ground squirrels were virtually annihilated; their bodies were found in attitudes characteristic of violent death by poisoning. Dead muskrats were found in the treated areas, dead rabbits in the fields. The fox squirrel had been a relatively common animal in the town; after the spraying it was gone.
>
> (p. 90)

Ironically, as Carson points out is often the case, the Japanese beetles, the targeted insect, seemed to be thriving—and continued their westward expansion—even after several years of spraying.

"Chemical death raining down": Aerial spraying

As if to placate, preemptively, a worried public, Carson says repeatedly that she is not entirely opposed to the use of chemical pesticides. What she *is* opposed to is the "automatic" resort to poisons to solve every problem, the "habit of killing" (p. 117) any time humans were even slightly inconvenienced by an unwanted animal or insect.

Because of this "habit," she argues, most use of pesticides was entirely without thoughtfulness or planning. She finds the lack of planning to mitigate their effect particularly enraging, because it seems so intentionally careless with life. She denounces the powers-that-be who don't examine whether pesticides are warranted and don't investigate the impact that pesticides would have beyond attacking the "pest" itself. This lack of curiosity is, in most instances, bureaucratized, Carson argues. Elected legislators and senior department officials refused to provide adequate funds to scientists in the civil service who might be in a position to study the effects of pesticides. In the case of the Japanese beetle eradication program in Illinois, for example, she was dismayed by the fact that although funds for chemical control came in seemingly never-ending streams, the biologists who tried to measure the damage to wildlife had to operate on a financial shoestring.

Carson is especially appalled by the wantonness of the killing, and the apparent bloodlust of some of the pesticide-pushers. In one remarkable paragraph, she demonstrates the disregard towards all life that she finds among the pesticide promoters:

> In a volume of Proceedings of one of the weed-control conferences ... I once read an extraordinary statement of a weed killer's philosophy. The author defended the killing of good plants "simply because they are in bad company." Those who complain about killing wildflowers along roadsides reminded him, he said, of antivivisectionists "to whom, if one were to judge by their actions, the life of a stray dog is more sacred than the lives of children."
> (p. 71)

What really enraged Carson, though, was the unthinking resort to *aerial* spraying of pesticides. Aerial spraying was the least precise way to apply poison. It was then, and it is now; we have now elevated one of the problems with aerial spraying to a term of art, "pesticide drift." Carson and her contemporaries knew about pesticide drift. She cites a 1947 article by F. Brooks with the unambiguous title, "The Drifting of Poisonous Dusts Applied by Airplanes and Land Rigs." She is scathing in her indictment of aerial spraying and the unquestioned assumption of bureaucrats, pesticide manufacturers and, increasingly, the public, that there was no alternative to aerial spraying. Have we fallen into a "mesmerized state," she wondered (p. 22).

Carson devotes a whole chapter to aerial spraying (Chapter 10, "Indiscriminately from the Skies"). Calling on Charles Elton's phrase, "the amazing rain of death," she railed against the folly of aerial spraying:

> Although today's poisons are more dangerous than any known before, they have amazingly become something to be showered down indiscriminately from the skies. Not only the target insect or plant, but anything—human or nonhuman—within range of the chemical fallout may know the sinister touch of the poison.
>
> (p. 141)

She went on to provide two case studies of the broad-spectrum killing left in the wake of aerial spraying: the fire ant eradication program, and the gypsy moth spraying program in Long Island.

The Long Island court case was particularly important to Carson as it was one of the catalysts for her interest in pesticides, and was one of the triggers that propelled her to write *Silent Spring*. In 1957 and 1958, much of Long Island was sprayed with pesticides as part of a vast east-coast gypsy moth eradication plan. The federal Department of Agriculture in the mid-1950s decided they would eradicate the gypsy moth on the entire east coast using DDT. In 1956, nearly a million acres were sprayed in the states of Pennsylvania, New Jersey, Michigan, and New York. Complaints of damage and reports of dying wildlife almost immediately ensued. As the pattern of the indiscriminate spraying of large areas seemed to be becoming more normalized, conservationists and worried citizens increasingly complained. When plans were announced for spraying 3 million acres in 1957, opposition became even stronger, and even more so when it became clear that urban areas were to be as indiscriminately sprayed as were forests. Long Island is a heavily populated region just east of New York City, consisting of many towns and suburbs, as well as salt marshes along the coasts; it came under the gun in 1957. The spray plan, organized by the combined federal and state Departments of

Agriculture, "showered down the DDT-in-fuel with impartiality." Dairy farms were under the spray path, and milk was contaminated; produce growers watched their crops wilt and die in the fields; beekeepers lost hundreds of hives with tens of thousands of bees. One beekeeper lost 400 colonies; another, 800 hives. In some cases, bee mortality within colonies was 100 percent. Fish ponds and salt marshes were sprayed. Birds, fish, crabs—all were killed with impunity. Anyone under the path of the daytime spraying—commuters and children alike—was drenched. A horse who drank from a water trough in a sprayed field was dead ten hours later. Cars were spotted with the oily mixture; flower gardens were destroyed.

But, as Carson continues, this was just the beginning of the litany of problems with the aerial attack. The spray plane pilots and companies were paid by the gallon rather than the acre—thus establishing a perfect incentive for multiple spray runs over the same area, and for heavy use of the DDT. Not all aerial spraying companies were properly registered or vetted; if problems ensued, as they did, the legal responsibility of unregistered companies was hard to establish.

In fact, it was the lawsuit filed against aerial spraying by several Long Island residents, eventually unsuccessful, that brought Carson into touch with Mary (Polly) Richards and Marjorie Spock—women who turned out to be enduring friends and allies. Spock and Richards, preparing for their legal case, had compiled a deep dossier of expert writings on pesticides, which they shared with Carson, becoming, as Lear says, a "chief clipping service" for Carson. The transcript of their trial was an invaluable resource for Carson.

Cry for the birds

Carson, an avid birdwatcher, was horrified by the wholesale massacre of birds by pesticides. In avian terms, one of the most important effects of Carson's book was the banning (*several* years after *Silent Spring*) of organochlorine pesticides—aldrin, DDT, and the like—in the United States and in much of the rest of the world.

Mostly, as Carson underscored, birds weren't the intended targets of pesticides, but, rather, they suffered the "collateral damage" of pesticide distribution. Birds are exquisitely vulnerable to pesticides:

many pesticides are granular, and attractive to birds who see them as seeds; many pesticides are designed to coat the outer shell or penetrate deeply into seeds; birds biomagnify the pesticides from their primary diet of worms, fish, or insects; birds are mobile over long distances and frequently, unwittingly, move into or through sprayed areas. The toll on birds is staggering—today, as in Carson's time. Today, an estimated 672 million birds are exposed annually to pesticides on US agricultural lands; of these, in any given year, 10 percent—67 million—are killed.[8] And that's just in the United States. This staggering number is a conservative estimate that takes into account only birds that inhabit farmlands, and only birds killed outright by ingestion of pesticides. The full extent of bird fatalities due to pesticides is extremely difficult to determine because most deaths go undetected. Carson was witnessing the very first years of this holocaust, and what she saw led her to despair—and action.

While birds mostly weren't the primary target of pesticides, sometimes they were. Carson reported on an example of farmers killing birds *en masse* with parathion in 1959. In southern Indiana, a group of farmers who were tired of blackbirds eating their corn decided to hire a spray plane to spray a nearby river system where the birds roosted. Rather than changing their agricultural practice (in favor of a corn variety with deep-set ears, not accessible to birds), the farmers "had been persuaded of the merits of poison" (p. 118), and set about to impose death on thousands of birds:

> The results probably gratified the farmers, for the casualty list included some 65,000 red-winged blackbirds and starlings. What other wildlife deaths may have gone unnoticed and unrecorded is not known. Parathion is not a specific for blackbirds: it is a universal killer. . . . rabbits or raccoons or opossums as may have roamed those bottomlands and perhaps never visited the farmers' cornfields were doomed.
>
> (p. 117)

Carson didn't flinch from describing the horrors of animals, especially birds, dying from pesticide poisoning. No doubt partly to shock her audience, and perhaps hoping to galvanize them into action, Carson spared few details.

Carson describes a 1959 Detroit campaign of spraying aldrin in an attack aimed at Japanese beetles. Spraying took place at various times of day, showering pellets of aldrin on people, playgrounds, lakes, and woods. The granules of poison accumulated on porches and sidewalks, and housewives swept them up like snow. The tiny granules lodged in roof shingles, eaves, and gutters and when it rained, the Michigan Audubon Society said, "every puddle became a death potion." She continues:

> Within a few days after the dusting operation, the Detroit Audubon Society began receiving calls about the birds . . . "The first . . . call I received on Sunday morning [was] from a woman who reported that coming home from church she saw an alarming number of dead and dying birds. The spraying there had been done on Thursday. She said there were no birds at all flying in the area, that she had found at least a dozen [dead] in her backyard and that the neighbors had found dead squirrels." Birds picked up in a dying condition showed the typical symptoms of insecticide poisoning—tremoring, loss of ability to fly, paralysis, convulsions.
> (pp. 87–88)

Following a shift in agricultural practices in England in 1959, to treat seeds with insecticides before sowing, dead birds piled up in fields and on streets:

> "The place is like a battlefield," a landowner in Norfolk wrote. "My keeper has found innumerable corpses, including masses of small birds—Chaffinches, Greenfinches, Linnets, Hedge Sparrows, also House Sparrows . . . the destruction of wild life is quite pitiful." . . . "Pigeons are suddenly dropping out of the sky dead," said one witness. Witnesses described huge bonfires on which the bodies of the birds were burned . . . of the [dead] birds analyzed, all but one contained pesticide residues . . . Along with the birds . . . [in six months] at least 1300 foxes died. Deaths were heaviest in the same counties from which sparrow hawks, kestrels, and other birds of prey virtually disappeared, suggesting that the poison was spreading through the food chain, reaching out from the seed eaters to the furred and feathered carnivores. The actions of the

moribund foxes were those of animals poisoned by chlorinated hydrocarbon insecticides. They were seen wandering in circles, dazed and half blind, before dying in convulsions.

(pp. 115–116)

From Sheldon, Illinois, Carson reports:

Scientific observers at Sheldon described the symptoms of a meadowlark found near death: "Although it lacked muscular coordination and could not fly or stand, it continued to beat its wings and clutch with its toes while lying on its side. Its beak was held open and breathing was labored." Even more pitiful was the mute testimony of the dead ground squirrels, which "exhibited a characteristic attitude in death. The back was bowed, and the forelegs with the toes of the feet tightly clenched were drawn close to the thorax . . . The head and neck were outstretched and the mouth often contained dirt, suggesting that the dying animal had been biting at the ground."

(pp. 94–95)

In outrage and agony, Carson asks, "By acquiescing in an act that can cause such suffering to a living creature, who among us is not diminished as a human being?" (p. 96).

Thematically and rhetorically, *Silent Spring* pivots around the birds. It is the "silencing" of birds by pesticides that gives the book its central trope. And it was a bird die-off from spraying that made Carson determined to write the book: in 1958, Olga Huckins wrote to Carson about the devastation of her backyard bird sanctuary in Duxbury, Massachusetts, by aerial spraying aimed at mosquitoes— that also killed off virtually all insects along with songbirds and bees. Huckins could get no satisfactory response to her complaints to the state, and she went public with her complaints, as well as sharing her dismay with Carson, with whom she was previously acquainted.

Carson opens the Acknowledgements to *Silent Spring* with a note of thanks to Olga Huckins:

In a letter written in January 1958, Olga Owens Huckins told me of her own bitter experience of a small world made lifeless, and so brought my attention sharply back to a problem with which I had long been concerned. I then realized I must write this book.

(p. ix)

The aquatic holocaust

Carson loved the sea. She understood both freshwater and salt water aquatic environments. She knew how they worked and she marveled at the "exquisite" ecosystems of water. While the tragedy of pesticides for birds occupied the central stage in Carson's telling, when describing the threat to marine life and whole aquatic ecosystems Carson seems to run short of adjectives. Her chapter on "Rivers of Death" is replete with reports of devastation, annihilation, and, everywhere, death. This chapter is perhaps where her ecosystem analysis is at its best. Carson describes in great detail the interrelationships between forests and freshwater rivers, and the cascade of destruction that follows when the forests are sprayed: insects die, the fish that eat the insects die (if they aren't already dead), the frogs that bury in the mud die, the dragonflies die, the snails die.

Carson provides close descriptions of the destruction wrought in one river basin by the spraying conducted in the Miramichi region of New Brunswick, Canada (as she wryly observes, to save the pulp and paper industry from the budworm). In 1954, aerial spraying of DDT was conducted over the forests of the northwest Miramichi River basin. The pilots were given no instructions about trying to avoid spraying the river itself, and it's not clear they could have done so even if so instructed. Within two days, salmon and brook trout were rising, dead, to the surface of the river, gasping their last breath. Flies, birds, gnats, fish larvae were all dead or dying within a remarkably short window after spraying. By the end of August, the entire year's spawn of salmon had been killed.

Carson saved her strongest language for the destruction she saw to the environment she knew best—the salt water shores, bays, marshes, and estuaries.

"Holocaust" was a word she used only once in the book, and she used it to describe the spraying of the salt marshes of eastern Florida: "The scene as described was a macabre picture—something that might have been created by a surrealist brush. The snails moved among the bodies of the dead fishes and the moribund crabs, devouring the victims of the death rain of poison" (p. 228).

"Carnage" (p. 135) she also used only once, again to describe a massive spraying of dieldrin in 1955 on about 2,000 acres of salt marshes in eastern Florida—an attempt to eliminate the larvae of the sandfly. The effect on life in the waters was catastrophic. Scientists from the Entomology Research Center of the State Board of Health surveyed the carnage after the spraying and reported that the fish kill was "substantially complete." Everywhere, dead fishes littered the shores.

What outraged Carson particularly was that, in her estimation, the devastation brought to aquatic environments by mostly land-based spraying was inevitable and predictable. With the undisciplined use of aerial spraying, and given the realities of runoff, contamination of waterways from land-based poison was all but inevitable. Fish, Carson says, are almost "fantastically sensitive to the chlorinated hydrocarbons" (p. 129) that then made up the largest share of insecticides. In discussing a 1950 disaster in a river system in Alabama, she observes sharply that the disastrous results could easily have been foreseen: what transpired there was that heavy summer rains washed the toxaphene insecticides the cotton farmers were using into the river system, and the heavier the rains, the more toxaphene the farmers applied.[9] In short order, a massive aquatic kill ensued.

Threats to water environments came, Carson said, from three main sources: runoff into both fresh and salt water from treated agricultural land; river systems collaterally sprayed when the surrounding forests were; and salt marshes and estuaries often intentionally sprayed against insects that harbor there. While Carson brought an ecosystem sensibility to the analysis of this problem, she also took care to discuss the damage to livelihoods and economies that ensued from pesticide campaigns that killed large numbers of animals. This economic relationship was most directly evident with the fisheries: the commercial fisheries, recreational fishing, and water-based recreation in general, that all suffered when ecosystems were degraded by poisoning.

While speaking for the animals, Carson kept a steady eye on the impacts on humans, both in terms of health and economy. However, while keeping an eye on both, Carson didn't really address the tension that underlay this dualism: that sometimes, in order to provide or protect a strong economy, pesticides are deemed to be necessary— to the considerable peril of animals. This is a central environmental tension with which we continue to struggle.

Pesticides today

In the United States today, five decades after Carson sounded the alarm, pesticides are ubiquitous. They are used to kill prairie dogs in Kansas, gophers in Utah, grasshoppers in North Carolina, snails in Alabama, mosquitoes in Texas, thrips in Georgia, mice in Massachusetts, rats in New York, dandelions in Maine, crabgrass in Virginia, potato blight in Idaho, thistles in Alaska, citrus canker in Florida, pond algae in Pennsylvania, ants in Colorado, termites in Louisiana, spiders in Ohio. While 75–80 percent of all pesticides in the United States are used in agriculture, 75–85 percent of US households have at least one pesticide product (Delaplane, 1996, p. 2; USEPA, 2011, p. 20). Many people, especially urbanites or suburbanites, may not think of themselves as owning pesticides, but if you use cockroach sprays or baits, insect sprays or lotions, mice or rat poisons, flea and tick sprays, pet collars, mold or mildew sprays, kitchen, laundry, and bath sanitizers, wood preservatives, weed killers, or certain swimming-pool chemicals, then you are most likely using pesticides.

As of 2012, the EPA has approved more than 1,200 pesticide active ingredient chemicals for use, more than 65,000 pesticide products registered,[10] and maintains an inventory of more than 84,000 chemicals in its Toxic Substances Inventory.[11] About 5.1 billion pounds of pesticide products are used each year in the United States, comprised of almost a billion pounds of active pesticide ingredients (USEPA, 2011, p. 10).[12] There are more than 100 producers of pesticides in the United States, and about 14,000 distributors (USEPA, 2011, p. 20). In 2013 in the state of New York, more than 14,000 pesticide products are registered for use; in Florida, it's just over 16,000 pesticide products; in Illinois, 13,000; in Michigan, almost 17,000.[13]

Although the United States is the world's single largest user of pesticides, pesticides are prominent worldwide in everyday life. In

2007, about 5.2 billion pounds of pesticide active ingredients were used worldwide (USEPA, 2011, p. 9). The world's six largest pesticide manufacturers are household names, even if they're not known primarily as pesticide producers: Monsanto, Syngenta, Bayer, BASF, Dow, and DuPont.

Against all this, it now seems quaint to worry, as Carson did in 1962, about the "200 chemicals that have been created for use in killing . . . pests" or the "500 new chemicals that annually find their way into use in the US alone . . . sold under several thousand brand names" (p. 18). But Carson's worries are still our own. Many of the most lethal of the chemicals Carson worried about are still our own. The cultural assumptions, the regulatory framework, and the vast gaps in knowledge to which Carson drew attention are still our own.

Humans—especially agricultural workers—are still being poisoned at an alarming rate by pesticides. Between 1998 and 2005, there were over 3,000 cases of "acute pesticide poisoning," including one fatality, among agricultural workers in the United States (Calvert et al., 2008); deaths and injuries in the rest of the world are even more common. A late 1990s study estimates that about 1 million people a year are killed or suffer chronic illnesses as a result of pesticide poisoning (EnviroNews Forum, 1999). Spectacular die-offs of animals and birds as a result of pesticide exposure remain a common occurrence. In 1995, insecticides in Argentina killed almost 5 percent of the total world's population of Swainson's hawks—a long-distance migratory bird. Over 150 bird "die-offs" in the United States, involving as many as 700 birds in a single incident, have been attributed to diazinon—an organophosphate insecticide commonly used for lawn care. In 1990, diazinon was classified as a restricted ingredient, and banned for use on golf courses and turf farms, marking the first time regulatory action has been taken specifically on behalf of birds; however, in most states, diazinon is still available over the counter for use on home lawns and parks, and as much as 10 million pounds of diazinon are still used yearly, primarily by home owners.[14]

Many of the most damaging and spectacular industrial accidents in the past few decades—in terms of human and animal health impacts and widespread environmental damage—have been related to pesticide production and use. Among them:

- The 1976 Seveso disaster: an explosion at the ICEMSA chemical plant, which was manufacturing pesticides near Seveso, Italy, resulted in the largest accidental release of dioxins known in the world. Hundreds of domestic and wild animals were immediately killed, with about another 80,000 animals eventually slaughtered to prevent contamination of the food chain. Long-term human health carcinogenic and reproductive health effects are still being tracked.

- The 1986 Sandoz chemical spill: a fire at an agrochemical warehouse in Switzerland owned by Sandoz, released tons of pollutants into the air, the soil, groundwater, and runoff into the Rhine river, resulting in massive mortality of all wildlife downstream and leaving enduring environmental damage.

- Bhopal, India, 1984: an explosion at a Union Carbide chemical plant producing pesticides in India, caused the world's worst chemical accident, killing over 3,000 people and injuring another 30,000, as well as killing thousands of animals.

And there are new problems, too, that Carson hadn't yet encountered—well beyond even her imaginings of the "dreams of the Borgias." Of particular note are genetically modified (GMO) crops, and the threat to bees.

Genetically modified crops

Since the mid-1990s, genetically modified agriculture has changed the relationship between agriculture and pesticides. One of the first modifications that GMO companies introduced was to produce herbicide-tolerant crops. Monsanto introduced the first, in 1996, with its "Roundup-ready" soybeans. What this meant was that the crop—in this case, soybeans—would survive being doused with herbicides—in this case "Roundup." The advantage of this was that farmers could easily kill weeds or unwanted plants in their fields while leaving their main crop untouched. Free from the fear of killing their prized crop, farmers, though, have been using more herbicides. And, in turn, weeds are developing resistance, which is leading to the use of even *more* herbicide. Several studies point to findings of increased herbicide use with GMO cropping: one researcher found that that GMO crops are driving up the volume of herbicide used each year by about 25 percent, and that, in the United States, the increase in the herbicides required to deal with tougher-to-control weeds on cropland planted to genetically modified crops has grown from 1.5 million pounds in 1999, to about 90 million pounds in 2011 (cited in Gilliam, 2012). Many of the older, higher-risk herbicides are being brought back to deal with the resistance problem. The GMO companies, such as Monsanto, say that the jury is still out, but most researchers say that this trend is unmistakable. In the United States, one of the bureaucratic arrangements that will make review and management of this problem more complicated is that the USDA regulates the crops while EPA regulates the herbicides.

The European Union has taken a strict regulatory stance towards GMO crops, in some measure because of concerns about this "pesticide treadmill" effect. European Union countries thus have, at different times, banned US food products that have been genetically modified; some members of Congress have joined the US farm lobbyists in efforts to end European Union bans.

Bees

Carson's descriptions of pesticide deaths of "bystander" insects include several reports of bee kills from pesticide spraying. But since Carson's time, the threat to bees has dramatically worsened. Modern agriculture depends largely on the services of bees as pollinators; about one-third of the crop species that are used in US agriculture rely directly on bees. Almost all flowering plants, including clover that dairy cows eat, depend on bees for their survival. And now, the bees are dying in large numbers, in mysterious ways, and with alarming speed. In one season alone—the winter of 2006–2007—more than a quarter of the bees in the United States died or disappeared—a mysterious syndrome that has been dubbed "colony collapse disorder" (CCD). Die-offs in much of Europe are at least as bad.

Many factors contribute—or could—to CCD, including the fact that bees have become the full-time workers for commercial pollinators and are often literally overworked, (perhaps "to death"), moved from farm to farm and region to region with less and less down time. But after intense scientific investigation, most scientists now agree that a new class of pesticides introduced in the 1990s called "neonicotinoids" is the primary culprit. Several studies concluded in 2012, pointed decisively to neonicotinoids as a central cause of bee die-offs. The French government has strictly limited the use of neonicotinoids; Germany and Italy followed suit; the European Union has imposed a temporary ban. In the United States, debate over regulating neonicotinoids has bogged down, as the manufacturers of neonicotinoids challenge the scientific findings, and the EPA process wheels turn slowly. Carson would be dismayed, but perhaps not surprised.

2012: A year of pesticide news

If you read the daily news, stories about pesticide mishaps and problems are commonplace. If you search the archives of any US media website for stories involving "pesticides," you'll come up with a surprising number of results. Just looking at *The New York Times* (NYT) and CNN news, for example, for 2012, yielded hundreds of stories.[15] This wasn't even a very sophisticated or extensive search—I didn't search, for example, for the more specific terms "herbicides" or "insecticides," nor for the broad category of "chemicals." The majority of the several hundred archived items I uncovered involved only a passing mention of "pesticide," and a few items were letters to the editors. Eliminating those, we're still left with more than 30 news reports centrally or mostly about pesticides. Some of the 2012 headlines were:

- NYT, December 11, 2012: "Pesticides: Now More Than Ever": A NYT columnist reviews recent studies that show that chronic exposure to pesticides is damaging not only to flora but to all creatures, including humans.

- NYT, December 8, 2012: "Argentina: Fire Forms Toxic Cloud": Buenos Aires' officials declared a public health emergency after a shipping container from China carrying a pesticide caught fire in the port, sending a thick, foul-smelling cloud of smoke over several parts of the city.

- CNN, December 4, 2012: "Pesticides in Tap Water, Produce Linked to Food Allergies": Pesticides in drinking water in the US may be playing a role in the prevalence of food allergies.

- CNN, October 17, 2012: "378 Peruvian Workers Sickened by Pesticide": Agricultural workers, mostly women, were sent to hospitals after inhaling a pesticide that had been sprayed a few hours earlier on an adjacent field.

- NYT, November 22, 2012: "Endangered and Targeted: Fight to Save Oriental Stork Captivates China": Hunters in China are increasingly using pesticides, especially the highly toxic carbofuran, to kill birds easily; they sell the meat to game restaurants.

- NYT, November 21, 2012: "Maker of Methyl Iodide Ends US EPA Registration": The maker of the controversial pesticide, methyl iodide, which is injected into the soil to kill insects and plant diseases, has removed all its products from the US market and will end all sales permanently.

- NYT, November 6, 2012: "As Dengue Fever Sweeps India, a Slow Response Stirs Experts' Fears": An epidemic of dengue fever is overwhelming the health system; neighborhoods in New Delhi are regularly sprayed with pesticides, but dengue continues to spread.

- CNN, October 13, 2012: "Indian Girl Seeks Justice After Gang Rape": The father of a 16-year-old girl who was raped in Haryana, India, fearful about the future for his daughter and distressed by the violence against his daughter, committed suicide by swallowing pesticides.

- NYT, September 21, 2012: "Honey Producers Lament a Bad Season for Bees": Honey production in parts of Europe is down as much as 90 percent; pesticide use is one factor in dramatic declines of bee colonies worldwide.

- NYT, September 20, 2012: "BASF Buys US Crop Chemicals Maker Becker Underwood": The world's largest chemicals maker, BASF, took over a US crop protection company.

- NYT, September 17, 2012: "In Conversation With: Investigative Reporter Sasha Chavkin": An interview with a reporter who has investigated clusters of chronic kidney disease in India; pesticides are a primary suspect.

- CNN, September 13, 2012: "Mysterious Tourist Deaths in Asia Prompt Poison Probe": A string of mysterious deaths of tourists in Thailand and Vietnam is tentatively tied to insecticides sprayed in the guest rooms and beds to kill bedbugs.
- NYT, September 7, 2012: "Scott's Miracle-Gro to Pay $12.5M Over Pesticides": Scott's, the world's largest maker of residential-use pesticides, pled guilty to illegally applying insecticides (that are toxic to birds) to its wild bird food products, falsifying pesticide registration documents, distributing pesticides with misleading and unapproved labels, and distributing unregistered pesticides.
- CNN, September 4, 2012: "Should You Buy Organic?": One of several stories about a controversial study that showed that people who ate organic food (which includes, of course, foods grown without pesticides), are not necessarily healthier nor do they live longer than those who don't. This was one of a flurry of stories that were prompted by this study.
- NYT, September 3, 2012: "Stanford Scientists Cast Doubt on Advantages of Meat and Produce": A study finds that conventional fruits and vegetables are not less nutritious than their organic counterparts, but they do have more pesticide residues.
- NYT, August 31, 2012: "City Has Sudden Jump in West Nile Cases": The city of New York has been spraying pesticides in sections of the city to reduce mosquito populations.
- CNN, August 20, 2012: "Pesticide Spraying Resumes in Dallas": A resurgence in West Nile virus throughout Texas has prompted pesticide spraying in many counties and towns, and has also prompted controversy about the spraying.
- CNN, August 15, 2012: "Pesticides Blamed for Massive Bird Deaths": A farmer in New Jersey used an approved pesticide, granular avitrol, on his fields; a massive bird

die-off resulted, and nearby residents were upset as birds dropped dead—literally—in their backyards and driveways.

- NYT, August 9, 2012: "LA Judge Dismisses Workers' Lawsuit Against Dole": A Superior Court judge dismissed a lawsuit brought by nearly 3,000 Filipino workers claiming injury from pesticide exposure while they worked for Dole Food Co. 30 years earlier.
- NYT, July 23, 2012: "New Paint Wipes Out Infestation in a Village": An experimental house paint that is impregnated with pesticides, tested in Bolivia, shows promise in eliminating mosquitoes and other pests.
- CNN, June 19, 2012: "Apples Bag Top Spot on Annual 'Dirty Dozen' List": Apples and celery topped the list of produce with the highest levels of pesticide residue. This prompted several other stories of the "how safe is your produce" variety.
- CNN, June 13, 2012: "Biologists, Volunteers Rush to Save Florida Butterfly Species": The once iconic Schaus swallowtail butterfly in southern Florida is nearing extinction; pesticide use is contributing to their decline.
- CNN, June 3, 2012: "Study: Bed Bug 'Bombs' Don't Work": Do-it-yourself "foggers" that fill rooms with aerosol insecticides, readily available and inexpensive, are not effective against bedbugs.
- CNN, June 8, 2012: "Make Your Garden Pet-Friendly": Warns against using pesticides in household gardens where domestic pets are likely to roam.
- CNN, May 23, 2012: "Official Says 'Natural' Causes Behind Dolphin Deaths in Peru": Officials said that hundreds of dead dolphins that washed up on Peruvian shores died of natural causes, not pesticide exposure, as was previously suggested.
- NYT, May 8, 2012: "Dead Dolphins and Birds are Causing Alarm in Peru": At least 877 dolphins and more than 1,500 birds, most of them brown pelicans and boobies, have died since the government began tracking the deaths in

February; the media and environmentalists think pesticides might be implicated.

- CNN, May 11, 2012: "The Mysterious Case of the Disappearing Bees": New studies link "colony collapse disorder" of bees with pesticide use.
- CNN, April 30, 2012: "Study: Common Pesticide Affects Developing Brain": A new study suggests that at even low doses, a common pesticide, Chlorpyrifos, may be subtly influencing brain development in children.
- NYT, April 25, 2012: "Dow Corn, Resistant to a Weed Killer, Runs into Opposition": Growing opposition to GMO corn developed by Dow, because with this corn farmers will then be able to use more herbicides to kill weeds without harming their corn crop.
- NYT, March 29, 2012: "Two Studies Point to Common Pesticide as a Culprit in Declining Bee Colonies": A class of pesticides called "neonicotinoids" is implicated in deaths of bees and collapses of bee colonies.
- NYT, March 21, 2012: "Maker Pulls Pesticide Amid Fear of Toxicity": The manufacturer of a methyl iodide soil fumigant, approved and intended for use in California's strawberry fields, voluntarily removed the product from the US market following concerns and controversy.
- CNN, February 28, 2012: "Chemical Factory Explosion in China Kills at Least 12": A factory in Hebei province that made pesticides exploded, killing several workers.
- NYT, February 3, 2012: "Man Admits to Selling Illegal and Dangerous Pesticides": A New York man was arrested for selling hundreds of packets of "unregistered and mislabeled" pesticides from China.
- CNN, January 27, 2012: "War of Words Over Looming EPA Dioxin Study": The EPA, which already classified dioxins as "likely carcinogens," is about to issue its long-awaited report on risks from dioxins. Dioxins are produced as by-products of pesticide manufacturing, among other industrial processes.

For further discussion/exploration

- Find out if your state or city uses pesticides to clear vegetation on highway roadsides, railway beds, and utility rights of way. When was that decision made, who are the decision-makers, and what public review of the policy is included (if any)?

- Make an inventory of pesticides that are in your home.

- In her arguments against pesticides, Carson names specific chemicals, but she doesn't name the names of any pesticide *manufacturers*. Do you think she should have? Would her arguments be strengthened or weakened if she had done so?

- If Carson were writing today, what environmental problem do you think she would identify as the most important? Would it still be pesticides?

- The banning of pesticides such as chlordane and DDT by the EPA, and their inclusion on the Stockholm Conventions' list of the 'dirty dozen' POPs seems to vindicate Carson. But most of these were not banned in the United States until 20–30 years *after Silent Spring*. Why did it take so long to act on what Carson and her scientific colleagues knew in the 1960s to be extremely dangerous chemicals? Do you think that local, national or international regulatory agencies should—or could—act any faster on dangers discovered today?

- Some critics say that bee die-offs are *not* due to pesticides. What alternative explanations are being offered? What do you think of the evidence for the various explanations?

- Why do you think the US government has not ratified the Stockholm Convention? What does the US government say about why it hasn't?

4

One in Every Four

Carson devoted four chapters in *Silent Spring* to matters of human health (Chapters 11 through 14). It was, perhaps, with these chapters that Carson struggled the most, both professionally and personally. She had been deep in the scientific literature, pushing herself to the frontier of scientific knowledge to knit together the complex medical and biological evidence she would reveal in these chapters when, in April 1960, after several health problems, her doctor told her she needed a radical mastectomy for "cysts" in her left breast. She was bent on keeping her health disruptions secret, and she told only her innermost circle of friends. She was a private person at the best of times, but on the brink of *Silent Spring* she was also aware that any news of her ailing health would cheer her critics: "I have no wish to read of my ailments in literary gossip columns. Too much comfort to the chemical companies," she wrote to Marjorie Spock after her April surgery (quoted in Lear, 2009, p. 367).

By the end of 1960, she discovered that her surgeon had misled her about the seriousness of the "cysts," and as she was finishing up the health chapters for *Silent Spring*, she came to know she was seriously ill with cancer. The fact that her surgeon purposely misled her was not unusual in the early 1960s. The women's health movement was still a decade away, and as Linda Lear points out, this deception would have been the "normal" patriarchal protocol between male doctors and female patients:

> Medical protocols between a single, female patient and her physician in the 1950s and 1960s might help explain why Sanderson [the doctor] had not told Carson the truth. Typically, in the case of

a married woman, the patient herself would not have been told she had a malignancy, but her husband, had he asked directly, would have been given the full account. But even these conventions do not explain why, knowing that the tumor had already metastasized, Sanderson failed to suggest further radiation treatment even as a precautionary measure. No explanation suffices except the possibility that he considered her cancer so far advanced that no treatment would make any difference in her life expectancy.

(Lear, 2009, p. 368)

In early 1961, breast cancer metastasis was discovered. Carson had radiation therapy, and an onslaught of serious health problems ensued, from ulcer flare-ups to a dangerous staph infection. She struggled to make informed health decisions for herself in the midst of incomplete medical information and contradictory advice—gold therapy or not? chemotherapy or not?—just as she was struggling with the evidence, incomplete and often tentative, on the health impacts of pesticides. Her inner and outer worlds were weirdly mirroring one another about how to assess assaults to health in the midst of uncertain or incomplete knowledge. By 1962, mere months before *Silent Spring* was published, Carson received unequivocal confirmation from her doctors that the cancer had spread and that the prognosis was grave. The closer she got to first release in *The New Yorker*, the more intent Carson was to hide her illness. There could be little doubt that public acknowledgement of her cancer would have undermined her credibility as an unbiased analyst of pesticides. Carson suffered grave health crises for the next year and a half, finally succumbing in April 1964 to a heart attack.

Carson left no record of whether she thought her own cancer might have had an environmental root—or if indeed she thought there was *any* knowable cause. But as an overall rubric, beyond the personal, Carson was convinced that environmental disruptions produced human health disruptions. At the time she published *Silent Spring*, she was one of the very few scientists to take such a sweeping view of interrelationships between human health and the environment.

In many ways, given Carson's knowledge of exquisitely balanced ecologies, how could she not make the leap to human health? But so few did. Carson was leading the way in her assertion of the direct interchange between external and internal environments. Some of the arguments were simply common sense—how could we imagine that drinking water poisonous enough to kill cattle and cats would not harm humans? How could we imagine that chemical burdens absorbed by birds would not also be burdens when absorbed in human bodies? Even today, with 50 years beyond Carson of science, wisdom, and observation, many environmentalists wryly observe that we are living as though we all have another planet to go to, some way to escape the consequences of our environmental actions. In 1950s America, the notion that humans could be limited by their environment, or were subject to the same ecological disruptions as other animals, was not only a new idea but a positively un-American one. Carson knew she would encounter strong headwinds.

Domesticating the poisons

In the 20 years between Carson's first employment at the Fish and Wildlife Service and her first crack at the book that would become *Silent Spring*, she witnessed the introduction of terrifyingly powerful synthetic chemicals and a dramatic rise in pesticide use, driven more by industrial competition and profits, as well as the scientific "thrill" of developing ever more powerful synthetic chemicals, than by an actual defined need for yet more pesticides.

Marketing pesticides to farmers was easy. The "need" for pesticides in the agricultural sector seemed self-evident—then, as now. But although farming represented a large sector of the American economy in the 1950s, the pesticide manufacturers had their eyes on another prize, just as big. They wanted to market pesticides to everyone, not just farmers. The newly affluent, expanding, suburbanizing, American middle class offered an irresistible opportunity. Americans had to be convinced to bring pesticides home.

Marketing pesticides for household use required their manufacturers to craft a three-prong approach: first, marketing lawn care to men, persuading them that good lawn care (as defined by the pesticide manufacturers) was a mark of good citizenship and manly responsibility; second, marketing to women on the basis that modern pesticides allowed them to protect their children from illnesses borne by insects, and marked *them* as caring mothers; and, third, marketing to both men and women (though mostly women) for gardening. The social history of the lawn and the making of modern mothering are topics beyond the scope of this book—and very good social histories on both are available[1]—but the campaign to bring pesticides into American households was a carefully contrived commercial campaign. (This campaign needs continual propping up: today, in the face of current anti-pesticide and anti-lawn campaigns, the pesticide industry has redoubled its efforts to ensure that homeowners don't relinquish their pesticides. One such current industry-led effort, "Debug the Myths," offers 1950-ish boosterism: "We know you can handle the truth— pesticides help keep our families healthy and our homes happy.")[2]

As soon as DDT was released from the military to the civilian market, manufacturers started their campaign to domesticate pesticides. A typical advertisement from *Women's Day* magazine in 1947, makes, to our modern sensibilities, a horrifying pitch: a photograph shows a typical, white, presumptively middle-class woman bending over a crib that holds a smiling baby, under the large-font banner "Protect Your Children Against Disease-Carrying Insects." "How is she to protect her infant?", the viewer might wonder. DDT-impregnated wallpaper! In Disney "Jack and Jill" or "Disney Favorites" patterns, no less. The copy says it is "effective against disease-carrying insects for one year" and promises that this DDT-impregnated wallpaper is "*certified* to be absolutely safe for home use."

This campaign was typical of its time—a direct appeal to the emerging middle class to demonstrate its commitment to family values and a safe modern life through embracing chemicals. Manufacturers of pesticides worked ceaselessly to persuade the American middle class that pesticides would protect their homes and usher their arrival into the American Dream. Carson notes with alarm that use of poisons in the home was made easy and attractive:

> Kitchen shelf paper, white or tinted to match one's color scheme, may be impregnated with insecticide, not merely on one but on

both sides . . . With push-button ease, one may send a fog of dieldrin into the most inaccessible nooks and crannies of cabinets, corners, and baseboards. If we are troubled by mosquitoes, chiggers, or other insect pests . . . we have a choice of innumerable lotions, creams, and sprays for application to clothing or skin. Although we are warned that some of these will dissolve varnish, paint, and synthetic fabrics, we are presumably to infer that the human skin is impervious to chemicals . . . an exclusive New York store advertises a pocket-sized insecticide dispenser, suitable for the purse or for beach, golf, or fishing gear. We can polish our floors with a wax guaranteed to kill any insect that walks over it. We can hang strips impregnated with the chemical lindane in our closets and garment bags or place them in our bureau drawers . . . All these matters attended to, we may round out our day with insecticides by going to sleep under a mothproof blanket impregnated with dieldrin.

(pp. 158–159)

Carson goes on to remark that government agencies gave their stamp of approval to domesticating the pesticides. *Home and Garden Bulletins* from the USDA, she remarks, regularly encouraged people to spray their clothing with oil solutions of DDT, dieldrin, chlordane, or any of several other moth killers.

As appalled as Carson is by the campaigns to make pesticides cozy and convenient, she is even more worried that these advertisements give no indication that these materials are dangerous. Carson says, for example, that the American Medical Association campaigned against lindane vaporizers, considering them highly dangerous—but the unaware consumer, lulled by advertisements for domestic and personal uses of pesticides, would know nothing of these controversies or dangers.[3]

While manufacturers were appealing primarily to women to keep their homes safe through the liberal use of pesticides, a campaign for the outdoors—designed to appeal primarily to men—was just as intense. Carson decried the "fad of gardening by poisons" (p. 160), and the slick advertising campaigns mounted to encourage consumers to bring pesticides home. The use of pesticides in and around the home was marketed as a sign of modernity and of middle-class obligation. Gardening, Carson says, is now linked with the super poisons that are available in every hardware store, supermarket, and garden center. With very little cautionary advice to consumers who are urged to buy deadly materials,

> a constant stream of new gadgets make it easier to use poisons on lawn and garden—and increase the gardener's contact with them. One may get a jar-type attachment for the garden hose, for example, by which such extremely dangerous chemicals as chlordane or dieldrin are applied as one waters the lawn . . . Besides the once innocuous garden hose, power mowers also have been fitted with devices for the dissemination of pesticides, attachments that will dispense a cloud of vapor as the homeowner goes about the task of mowing his lawn.
> (p. 159)

Carson was dismayed by the trivial uses for pesticides. She remarked caustically on the role of advertising and the manipulation of class (and gender) identity by pesticide manufacturers in their effort to mount a campaign against crabgrass on suburban lawns. She and Betty Friedan, who was at the same moment writing her book *The Feminine Mystique* about the ways distinctive suburban masculinities and femininities were forged, might have had much to say to one another. They were both writing about the toxicities of suburbia, although from different perspectives. Carson literally so:

> The mores of suburbia now dictate that crabgrass must go at whatever cost. Sacks containing chemicals designed to rid the lawn of such despised vegetation have become almost a status symbol. These weed-killing chemicals are sold under brand names that never suggest their identity or nature. To learn that they contain chlordane or dieldrin one must read exceedingly fine print placed on the least conspicuous part of the sack.
> (p. 161)

Carson was amazed that anyone could walk into a store and purchase, without any question or registration or permit required, death-dealing chemicals. In her 1963 testimony before a Congressional committee, she implored lawmakers to restrict the sale and purchase of pesticides "at least to those capable of understanding the hazards and following directions . . . We place much more stringent restrictions on the sale of drugs—[a man made ill by spraying] could buy the chemicals that made him ill with no restrictions, but had to have prescriptions to buy the drugs to cure him" (Carson, 1963, p. 13).

The manufacturers were astonishingly successful in persuading Americans to bring pesticides home. The American home-and-garden sector today, 50 years after *Silent Spring*, consumes about 70 million pounds of active pesticide ingredients a year, and accounts for almost one-quarter of all pesticide use in the United States; of all *insecticides*, it accounts for 38 percent (USEPA, 2011, p. 6). The most common pesticide used on home gardens (as a lawn weed killer, used in over 1,500 pesticide products) is 2,4-D—a pesticide that Carson warned about in 1962. In *Silent Spring*, Carson warned of several cases of people who had suffered neuritis or paralysis after 2,4-D exposure. Carson also worried that there was sufficient evidence to suspect that 2,4-D mimicked the chromosome damage that radiation can cause at a cellular level, interrupting the oxidation of cells.

Today, more than 50 years and millions of pounds of its use later, considerable controversy still swirls around the possible health effects of 2,4-D, with some activist groups drawing attention to studies that link 2,4-D to elevated rates of non-Hodgkin's lymphoma; most public health authorities and the manufacturers of 2,4-D contest this finding. Nonetheless, the State of New Jersey's current official "hazardous substance fact sheet" for 2,4-D, for example, identifies these possible health effects from exposure to it (State of New Jersey, 2008; emphasis as in original):

- 2,4-D can affect you when inhaled and by passing through the skin.
- 2,4-D should be handled as a CARCINOGEN – WITH EXTREME CAUTION.
- 2,4-D may cause reproductive damage. HANDLE WITH EXTREME CAUTION.
- Contact can irritate the skin and eyes.

- Inhaling 2,4-D can irritate the nose and throat.
- Inhaling 2,4-D may irritate the lungs. Higher exposures may cause a build-up of fluid in the lungs (pulmonary edema), a medical emergency.
- Higher or repeated exposure may damage the nerves causing headache, muscle weakness, and poor coordination in the arms and legs.
- 2,4-D can cause nausea, vomiting, diarrhea and abdominal pain.
- 2,4-D may damage the liver and kidneys.

Manufacturers would perhaps argue that these are the outer limits of possible reactions—and uncertain, thus the careful use of the word "may." But the operative concern for the public is that for 2,4-D, as for most of the pesticides in use today, as in Carson's time, we *don't* really know the health effects—chronic, acute, or merely "possible."

In the United States, the primary regulatory agency for pesticides— the EPA—is underfunded and understaffed to the extent that it can't monitor and regulate pesticides (nor the tens of thousands of other chemicals) as effectively as the public assumes they do. In a 1986 study of nonagricultural pesticide regulation, the US Government Accountability Office (GAO)—the government's watchdog agency— determined that:

> The pesticide industry sometimes makes safety claims for its products that EPA considers to be false or misleading.
> We found that the general public receives misleading information on pesticide hazards and that EPA had taken few civil penalty enforcement actions against such claims. We concluded that EPA had made limited use of its authority over unacceptable advertising safety claims and recommended that it take steps to strengthen and improve its program for controlling such claims.
> (GAO, 1990, p. 8)

In a 1990 follow-up, the GAO found few improvements in the intervening years, and they asserted that it was still the case that pesticide manufacturers were making false claims about the safety or nontoxicity of their products (GAO, 1990, p. 12). The EPA, the GAO discovered, had very little certain evidence about the health effects of the most commonly used pesticides. Almost 20 years later, in 2009, the GAO asserted baldly that the EPA lacked adequate scientific information on the toxicity of most chemicals used commercially in the United States, and that its health risk database was all but obsolete (GAO, 2009). Carson would recognize this debilitating pattern and would be dismayed that it has so stubbornly persisted.

Life just not quite fatal

Carson, 50 years earlier, was overwhelmed both by the growing ubiquity of pesticides and by how little was known about their effects. It was this juxtaposed tension that compelled her forward even during the many times, as her biographers recount, that she felt she could not write *Silent Spring*. Her passion is evident in the opening paragraphs of Chapter 3, "Elixirs of Death." For the first time in human history, she warns, every human being lives in a man-made chemical fog. From the moment of conception (not just birth) until death, she says, humans encounter synthetic chemicals everywhere and all the time. In the less than two decades (when Carson was writing) of their invention and release into the world, synthetic chemicals have become truly ubiquitous:

> They have been recovered from most of the major river systems and even from streams of groundwater flowing unseen through the earth. Residues of these chemicals linger in soil to which they may have been applied a dozen years before. They have entered and lodged in the bodies of fish, birds, reptiles, and domestic and wild animals so universally that scientists carrying on animal experiments find it almost impossible to locate subjects free from such contamination. They have been found in fish in remote mountain lakes, in earthworms burrowing in soil, in the eggs of birds—and in man himself. For these chemicals are now stored in the bodies of the vast majority of human beings, regardless of

age. They occur in the mother's milk, and probably in the tissues of the unborn child.

(p. 24)

Carson muses that we have fallen into a mesmerized state that ecologist Paul Shepard, describes as "life with only its head out of water, inches above the limits of toleration of the corruption of its own environment." Shepard continues, "Why should we tolerate a diet of weak poisons, a home in insipid surroundings, a circle of acquaintances who are not quite our enemies, the noise of motors with just enough relief to prevent insanity? Who would want to live in a world which is just not quite fatal?" (cited in Carson, p. 22).

She invokes, again, the notion that an authoritarian force has brought us to this brink. This dystopia, she argues throughout *Silent Spring*, is the product of an almost fanatical zeal in the pest-control community (by which she means private industry as well as government agencies) who press forward ruthlessly in quest of a sterile world.

Throughout *Silent Spring*, Carson offers up many explanations for the forces that pressed this world on us: our "inattention" (p.118); the hubris that humans could own and control nature; the imperative of profits; the contrivance of false assurances, outright deception, and the corruption of the regulatory–industry relationship; the "allure" of militarized power; the insensate logic of science; blindness to the wonders of nature; wishful thinking; fascination with "the new"; lack of knowledge, including willful lack of knowledge; bureaucratic parsimony with resources that might enable us to find out more about the real dangers; and a failure of imagination, among others.

Carson might have been interested in contemporary analyses of risk-taking that focus on the social construction of masculinity. Prompted largely by an examination of the behaviors that caused the global financial crisis of 2008—another opportunity to ask big questions about how we were brought to a brink—many analysts have been exploring the possibility that there are alignments between certain forms of masculinity and risk tolerance, especially an unreasonable willingness to create and take high-risk stakes.[4] Carson didn't bring a feminist analysis to *Silent Spring*, but she had an open mind and a real drive to understand how we had gotten ourselves into the position of creating the "just not quite fatal" world. She might have been intrigued by these analyses.

Poison on the plate

Carson well understood that severe exposure and acute health reactions to pesticides, including immediate deaths, were not common experiences for most people. Thus she was even more concerned with revealing the stealthy health impacts—the everyday exposures to pesticides—that would, over time, accumulate. It was not intuitively apparent to most people that an onset of illness, perhaps for many people occurring later in life when health problems might be expected, could be the result of pesticide exposure. Pesticides were becoming so common in everyday life that Carson knew that pesticide exposures for most people were diffuse and chronic, and spread over a lifetime, and were thus hard to "prove" dangerous. But she also knew they were.

Carson knew that the real dangers of pesticides were to be found not so much in the acute, high-dose, one-time (often accidental) exposures, but in the everyday, chronic, lower-level exposures. Attention to the chronic and low-level effects of exposure to toxic materials has often been contested territory. For example, Alice Stewart, a British epidemiologist, and contemporary of Carson's, was one of the only scientists sounding the alarm about chronic and low-level exposure to radiation. In the late 1950s, Stewart proved that X-raying pregnant women could cause considerable damage to fetuses. (It's thanks to Stewart that every woman is now asked whether she's pregnant "or could be" whenever she goes in for even the most routine X-ray, whether for a fractured finger or bruised hip.) Her research was, at first, attacked and dismissed. In the 1970s, Stewart shocked the scientific world with evidence of high rates of cancers among employees at nuclear facilities, starting with the Hanford (USA) plutonium production facility.[5] Stewart's work on X-ray exposures and on chronic nuclear plant radiation exposure was widely dismissed at the time—and *she* was attacked, also, as an overwrought woman alarmist—even though in almost all instances she has subsequently proven to be exactly right and prescient. But there is something about work on "low-level" and "chronic" environmental health processes that often provokes knee-jerk hostility and dismissive responses from mainstream medical and industrial interests. This dynamic may be slowly shifting, but for scientists such as Stewart and Carson, to focus on "low-level" exposures put them on the maligned far edges of mainstream environmental and medical research.

Carson builds the case against low-level chronic pesticide exposures methodically in the first of the four chapters devoted to health. The contamination of the environment and all living things therein is not, she says, simply a consequence of mass spraying. For most people, Carson says, acute exposure events seldom happen. Instead, for most of us, our exposure to toxic chemicals is a daily event, a birth to death immersion in a chemical fog. Carson is determined that her readers understand that the accumulation of small insults produces a progressive build-up and a cumulative poisoning.

Having in previous chapters worked her way through the chemistry of the most common pesticides, and introduced readers to notions of persistence, bioaccumulation and biomagnification, Carson was ready to pull those ideas together to paint a portrait of the health dangers of pesticides. To launch her discussion, she reminds readers of some of the key points:

- pesticides persist in the environment for decades; this means one doesn't need to have been present at the moment of spraying to be exposed;
- in the body, many pesticides are stored in fat, where they can reside for years;
- being at the top of the food chain means that humans eat the pesticides that every animal lower on the food chain themselves eats or the pesticides that every vegetable is exposed to in the soil.

Carson worked through the medical reports, available even then, that DDT residues had been found in virtually every member of the general population, even those with no known gross exposure to insecticides. How, then, she asks rhetorically, had the DDT come to be present in everyone's body?

The answer was: Food.

Carson told a shocked audience that food was the most common pathway of poison into the human body and that the "fact that every meal we eat carries its load of chlorinated hydrocarbons is the inevitable consequence of the almost universal spraying or dusting of agricultural crops with these poisons" (p. 163). Carson acknowledged that the question of the presence—and significance—of chemical residues in foods was hotly contested. Chemical manufacturers tended to either deny that residues existed, or to downplay their significance. Carson ruefully remarked that people who drew attention to the problem of food residues were quickly branded as fanatics or "cultists" who were seeking unreasonable purity in the food chain. Nonetheless, Carson was not to be deterred by anticipated criticism, and she laid out the scant evidence that, even in the late 1950s, pointed to a considerable public health concern.

Carson reports on a US Public Health (USPH) Survey that took samples from restaurant and institutional meals. Every food sample in the USPH survey contained DDT, some in enormous quantity. In a separate USPH sample of prison meals, some stewed fruits contained almost 70 parts per million of DDT, and some bread more than 100 parts per million. But, lest a reader think that her food—prepared lovingly and carefully at home—is safe, Carson warns that in the diet of the average American, meats or any products derived from animal fats contain heavy residues of chlorinated hydrocarbons—chemicals that are soluble in fat. While fruits and vegetables tend to have lower levels of residues, she points out that any such residues can't be removed by washing or cooking. There was little effective regulatory protection. Under Food and Drug regulations, no pesticide residues were allowed in milk—yet residues were always found in samples.

> [Residues] are heaviest in butter and other manufactured dairy products. A check of 461 samples of such products in 1960 showed that a third contained residues, a situation which the Food and Drug Administration characterized as "far from encouraging."
>
> (pp. 161–162)

Carson anticipated that readers would exclaim "But doesn't the government protect us from such things?" To which she replied, more or less, "Not much!" Carson then spends the rest of the chapter explaining the regulatory system that controlled pesticides on foods, and identifying its inadequacies.

In brief, this regulatory system, Carson explains, required the FDA to be responsible for monitoring and regulating pesticide residues. It did so through two basic regulatory processes:

a) The FDA set "tolerances"—maximum levels of allowable pesticide contamination—for a wide range of foods and a wide range of pesticides. The FDA set the tolerance level by reviewing pesticide manufacturers' laboratory tests on animals, which recorded the effects of pesticide exposure or ingestion on the animals at different exposure or ingestion levels—usually until the "LD-50" threshold was reached. Typically, the manufacturers used "LD-50" tests to determine the point at which the substance becomes acutely toxic: that is, they feed the poison to lab animals until a lethal dose (LD) was reached for 50 percent of their test animals (i.e. 50 percent of them die). The FDA worked backwards from these laboratory results to set a much lower level of "acceptable" food residue of the pesticide than the level that produced discernible ill effects on animals.

b) On a rotating basis, the FDA tested samples of foods for pesticide residues and would investigate—and sometimes remove supplies from the food chain—when higher-than-tolerance residues were found.

Carson pulls no punches in describing this as a counterintuitive system of food safety regulation in its conceptualization, as well as being ineffectual in its execution. She says that to set tolerances is "in effect, then . . . to authorize contamination of public food supplies with poisonous chemicals in order that the farmer and the processor may enjoy the benefit of cheaper production—then to penalize the consumer by taxing him to maintain a policing agency to make certain that he shall not get a lethal dose" (p. 165). She describes this system as astonishingly ineffective and morally bankrupt—an Alice in Wonderland topsy-turvy world.

Not only did Carson think that this system of tolerances-and-samples was balanced on upside-down priorities, a large part of her disdain for this system was based on a realistic understanding of the problems of implementing even this inadequate system. As she carefully details:

- "Tolerances" were often negotiated as a legal and practical matter between regulatory agencies and the manufacturers: political considerations intervened, there were few purely "health-based" tolerance levels set; tolerances were often set before complete testing (and field-based testing) results were available, and chemicals were released to market with a fast-track tolerance level (that often then had to be withdrawn later, but only after several years of use of the chemical in the food supply);

- It wouldn't be possible to set "purely health-based" tolerances in any event because so little was known about many of the chemicals;

- The FDA was outmanned and understaffed. It couldn't keep up with the flow of new chemicals;

- Because of the understaffing, the FDA tested only an infinitesimally small sample of the food supply; it also only had authority over food that was shipped in interstate commerce (any foods produced and sold within a single state were beyond its regulatory reach).

The food safety system that is in place *today*, is not much different than the system Carson excoriated 50 years ago.[6] In fact, in some ways, it might even be worse because so many regulatory agencies are involved; in 2007, the GAO called the American food safety oversight system "fragmented" and "inconsistent."[7] The EPA now sets the tolerances for pesticide residue levels on foods (it took over this responsibility from the FDA when it was founded); the "acceptable" tolerance level determined by the EPA is still based mostly on manufacturer laboratory animal tests; the food supply is tested by the USDA, which performs samples of foods for residues; the pesticide tolerances set by the EPA are enforced by the FDA, which also monitors domestically produced and imported foods traveling in interstate commerce (except meat, poultry, and some egg products, which are the responsibility of the USDA). Government regulatory agencies remain understaffed and underfunded. Sampling of foods in the supply chain is based on a rotating roster of small samples. And most chemicals found as residues on foods are not yet fully evaluated.

A 2009 GAO report on the EPA's capacity to regulate the toxicity of chemicals, found deep inadequacies:

> The EPA lacks adequate scientific information on the toxicity of many chemicals that may be found in the environment . . . Scientific information on the toxicity of chemicals is needed to, among other things, support effective and informed decision-making on whether EPA should establish controls to protect the public . . . EPA's inadequate progress in assessing toxic chemicals significantly limits the agency's ability to fulfill its mission of protecting human health and environment . . . [many safety assessments take too long], some of the assessments that have been in progress the longest cover key chemicals likely to cause cancer or other significant health effects. For example, EPA's assessment of dioxin has been underway for 18 years. The Assistant Administrator for Research and Development recently told a Congressional committee that the agency is years away from completing the dioxin assessment . . . Although dioxin is a known cancer-causing chemical to which humans are regularly exposed by eating such dietary staples as meats, fish, and dairy products, actions to protect the environment will likely be delayed until the assessment is complete. Since EPA estimates that the assessment process for complex chemicals such as dioxin could take 6 to 8 years, the public in the meantime will likely remain at risk.
>
> (GAO, 2009, pp. 22–23)

Food residues today

The findings of the food residue monitoring system—partial as they are, and as inadequate as the system is—are stunning. The USDA publishes an annual report of the results of its sampling of food for pesticide residues. Its 2011 report offers fascinating reading. For example, residues of 2,4-D were found in 41 percent of school or daycare well-water samples and in 60 percent of treated drinking-water samples from municipal systems, but none at levels that exceed regulatory tolerances; also "below tolerances" were the insecticide residues (bifenthrin) found in 38 percent of the green beans baby food samples, the fungicide (fludioxonil) found on 81 percent of plum samples, and the herbicide residues (glyphosate) found on 96 percent of soybeans sampled. Almost 40 percent of the cherry tomato samples had residues of three or more pesticides, as did 50 percent of the sweet bell peppers, as did 64 percent of the processed baby food pears samples (USDA, 2011).

A nonprofit group, the Environmental Working Group, puts out an annual "Dirty Dozen" list based on the USDA reports of the produce with the greatest pesticide residues. In 2010, the Dirty Dozen, with residues of 47–64 pesticides detected per serving, consisted of: celery, peaches, strawberries, apples, domestic blueberries, nectarines, sweet bell peppers, spinach, kale and collard greens, cherries, potatoes, imported grapes, and lettuce.[8]

The FDA publishes an annual report on pesticide residues found in common foods.[9] It uses a "market basket" approach—buying representative foods that an average American consumer might purchase. It then prepares these foods as the consumer might (washing vegetables and fruit, for example), but performs no other special handling. It then tests these foods for residues of about 300 chemicals. Its most recently available report (for 2009) reveals that many of the long-banned pesticides such as DDT and dieldrin remain circulating in the food system. Low levels of residues of DDT were found in 22 percent of the more than 1,000 foods sampled in the study; dieldrin in 9 percent. (This is not because DDT is being used illegally—when Carson foreshadowed the persistence of pesticides in the environment, even she would most likely not have anticipated detectable levels of banned pesticides after 40 years.)

As Carson identified, the bogged down regulatory process, caused in part by the ability of manufacturers to challenge regulations, to launch appeals, to delay action, and to lobby for favorable action, was then—and is now—a danger to the public. Carson put it bluntly, that the public was a guinea pig for chemicals. The regulatory system moved so slowly, Carson comments, that the public can be exposed to known carcinogens for years before effective regulations are in place: "[W]hat the public is asked to accept as 'safe' today may turn out tomorrow to be extremely dangerous" (p. 119). Carson tells the story of a particular (though unnamed) new pesticide that was introduced in 1955. The manufacturer—having killed the requisite number of laboratory animals—applied for a tolerance level that would allow for a low level of acceptable residues on any crops that may be sprayed. Scientists at the FDA thought that the lab test results showed that this chemical had carcinogenic properties, and they recommended zero tolerance (which would have prevented foods with residues being shipped across state lines). But the manufacturer appealed and brought considerable legal pressure to bear. In the ensuing negotiations, a "compromise" was reached: a tolerance of 1 part per million was to be established and the product marketed for two years, during which time further laboratory tests were to determine whether the chemical was actually a carcinogen. Carson finds this appalling, essentially positioning the public to be a guinea pig for chemical experimentation.

The ecology of the body

Carson was ahead of her time in extraordinary ways, nowhere more evident than in her explication of the health impacts of pesticides. She anticipated two of the paradigms that we now think of as being on the cutting edge of medical research: the health consequences of synergistic effects, and cumulative effects. Carson laid out these concerns in 1962:

   a) synergistic effects: that the real threat from chemical hazards in the body is the *synergy* of several or many chemicals; and

b) cumulative effects: that the human body accumulates a "body burden" of chemicals over time, and this total burden is what, in the end, manifests as disease or disruption.

Carson introduced a new paradigm: the "ecology of the body." This was an extraordinary leap for a writer in the early 1960s. To Carson, it seemed inescapably obvious that human health and the health of the environment were intertwined. This followed from her certainty that humans were not separate from nature, and that humans were subject to the same laws and perturbations and disruptions as other animals in the natural world. Nonetheless, to carry that framework into the human body was an extraordinary insight—an insight that the scientific and medical world is just now catching up to:

> There is also an ecology of the world within our bodies. In this unseen world minute causes produce mighty effects; the effect, moreover, is often seemingly unrelated to the cause, appearing in a part of the body remote from the area where the original injury was sustained. "A change at one point, in one molecule even, may reverberate throughout the entire system to initiate changes in seemingly unrelated organs and tissues," says a recent summary of the present status of medical research.
> (p. 170)

Carson makes the point that, given this "ecological" effect, the manifestation of disease may occur at considerable distance, in time and space, from the encounter with the poison that sets in motion the chain of molecular reaction. The person who is made ill by environmental exposures will have a very hard time tracing back the pathways of exposure and the disease outcome.

Synergistic effects

It is only in the past decade that the EPA has started to incorporate assessments of the synergistic effects of chemicals into *some* of its regulatory assessments—and even this early foray takes the EPA to the far limits of modern science, and presses against the limits of their budget and bureaucratic capacity. While it is impossible to anticipate and assess the impacts of the literally thousands of possible combinations of chemicals that we are exposed to throughout our lifetimes, the EPA is starting with some of the most common combinations. But this work is barely under way.

Carson understood the impossibility of tracking all of the combinations of chemicals, which was part of her larger argument against the proliferation of chemicals in everyday use. And she was well aware—and was one of the only scientists making this point in the 1960s—that the impact of exposure to multiple chemicals was more than just the sum of its parts. But, first, she might say, the parts had to be summed!

Carson makes the point that given the ubiquity of chemicals in post-war modern life, no one was exposed merely to a single chemical at only one time in some pure or isolated form. This was all the more true because chemicals accumulated in the fat tissues of the human body, so exposures to multiple chemicals didn't have to happen at the same time to produce synergistic effects. Carson also understood that true synergy meant that multiple chemicals magnified the effects of one another.

Carson relates the findings of a small FDA study conducted in the late 1950s that showed that when malathion (an organophosphate insecticide) was administered to laboratory animals in combination with other organic phosphates, a "massive poisoning" (p. 38) resulted—up to 50 times as severe as would have been predicted on the basis of simply summing up the two separate toxicities. In other words, 1/100th of the LD of each compound became fatal when the two were combined. The FDA tested other combinations, and in each case found that pairs of organic phosphates were orders of magnitude more toxic than their separate toxicities would predict. Carson explains that the toxicity is increased, or "potentiated," through the combined action—typically because one compound destroys the liver enzyme that is responsible for detoxifying the other!

> The two need not be given simultaneously. The hazard exists not only for the man who may spray this week with one insecticide and next week with another; it exists also for the consumer of sprayed products. The common salad bowl may easily present

a combination of organic phosphate insecticides. Residues well within the legally permissible limits may interact . . . [Further] the toxicity of an organic phosphate can be increased by a second agent that is not necessarily an insecticide. For example, one of the plasticizing agents may act even more strongly than another insecticide to make malathion more dangerous.

(pp. 38–39)

Carson was worried specifically about exposure to multiple chemicals through food and water. Just as the innocuous salad bowl might contain an unpredictable mix of pesticides, given the ubiquitous chemical pollution of the nation's waterways, Carson posits that a simple glass of water could contain a chemical mix that "no responsible chemist would think of combining in his laboratory" (p. 49). Even innocuous chemicals, when combined in unpredictable ways, can become lethal. And it's not only pesticides or agrochemicals that get combined in food and water. What, she asks, of the combination of chemicals and radioactive wastes that are discharged into waterways at increasing volumes?

In speaking about the inadequacies of the "tolerances" system of regulation, Carson makes the point clearly that synergistic effects are even more dangerous—and entirely unregulated:

Even if 7 parts per million of DDT on the lettuce in his luncheon salad were "safe," the meal includes other foods, each with allowable residues, and the pesticides on his food are, as we have seen, only a part, and possibly a small part, of his total exposure. This piling up of chemicals from many different sources creates a total exposure that cannot be measured. It is meaningless, therefore, to talk about the "safety" of any specific amount of residue.

(p. 165)

She extends this argument in a later section, again arguing that a single dose of a toxic chemical fed to a laboratory animal in a controlled experiment has little bearing on human experience. Humans are never exposed to one chemical alone. And just as unpredictable interactions can occur in a river system, so they can occur in the bloodstream of a person: "Whether released into soil or water or a man's blood, these unrelated chemicals do not remain segregated; there are mysterious and unseen changes by which one alters the power of another for harm" (p. 175).

In a 1963 statement before a Congressional committee, Carson explained to lawmakers that the scale of unknown synergistic effects of pesticides with one another, with other chemicals, and with radiation, was producing an environment of deadly interactions, most of which were impossible to measure or predict:

> The problem of pesticides can be properly understood only in context, as part of the general introduction of harmful substances into the environment. In water and soil, and in our own bodies, these chemicals are mingled with others, or with radioactive substances. There are little understood interactions and summations of effect. No one fully understands, for example, what happens when pesticide residues stored in our bodies interact with drugs repeatedly taken. And there are some indications that detergents, which are often present in our drinking water may affect the lining of the digestive tract so that it more readily absorbs cancer-causing chemicals. In attempting to assess the role of pesticides, people too often assume that these chemicals are being introduced into a simple, easily controlled environment as in a laboratory experiment. This, of course, is far from true.
>
> (Carson, 1963, p. 2)

Knowledge of the synergistic effects of the chemical soup that comprises our everyday environment still eludes both contemporary science and regulation. Sandra Steingraber, writing in 1997, picks up Carson's concern with synergistic effects of chemicals:

> The widespread introduction of suspected chemical carcinogens into the human environment is itself a kind of uncontrolled experiment. There remains no unexposed control population to whom the cancer rates of exposed people can be compared. Moreover, the exposures themselves are uncontrolled and multiple. Each of us is exposed repeatedly to minute amounts of

many different carcinogens and to any one carcinogen through many different routes. From a scientific point of view, such combinations are especially dangerous because they have the capacity to do great harm while yielding meaningless data. Science loves order, simplicity, the manipulation of a single variable against a background of constancy. The tools of science do not work well when everything is changing all at once.

(Steingraber, 1997, p. 29)

Cumulative effects

One of Carson's central arguments about human health effects of pesticides is that the impacts of exposure are only sometimes immediate and obvious. More typically, Carson would say, the effects are slow and reflect an accumulation of exposures over many years. She makes the point that most of us are accustomed to cause-and-effect being more closely related in both time and space. But if one understands that chemicals literally accumulate in the human body, and that damage to the integrity of cells or organs can also accrete over time, then this more conceptually complicated relationship makes sense. These slower, less tangible relationships are central to Carson's notion of the ecology of the body.

Carson doesn't use the phrase "body burden," as we might now, but her explanation of the damage from pesticide exposure through body *storage* of chemicals and the *accumulation* of chemicals prefigures that notion. Just as pesticides persist in the environment, Carson argues that they persist in the human body too, only to emerge as disease at some unknown future time.

Starting with even the smallest intake of DDT, she says, can produce a massive body burden. DDT is stored in the fatty tissues of the body, which then biomagnifies it by 100 times or more. Carson understands that the average reader would not be able to comprehend the scale of concern about residues—one or two "parts per million" sounds very small, to the average person on the street. Yes, she says, this *sounds* small, but the toxicity of these substances should not be underestimated. She reports the findings of DDT studies that show that 3 parts per million has been found to inhibit an essential enzyme in heart muscle; only 5 parts per million has caused cell death or disintegration of liver cells; and only 2.5 parts per million of the closely related chemicals dieldrin and chlordane did the same.

Carson points to some of the scientific debates raging about DDT, including over the question of whether there is a "floor" of exposure, below which DDT is not absorbed in the human body, or a "ceiling"—a maximum level of uptake—above which all excess DDT is excreted. Carson finds these arguments to be, largely, unimportant:

> According to various studies, individuals with no known exposure (except the inevitable dietary one) store an average of 5.3 parts per million to 7.4 parts per million; agricultural workers 17.1 parts per million; and workers in insecticide plants as high as 648 parts per million! So the range of proven storage is quite wide and, what is even more to the point, the minimum figures are above the level at which damage may begin.
>
> (pp. 29–30)

For comparison, by the late 1990s, the global average of levels of DDT in humans had declined to just below 7 parts per million.[10]

Medical investigation of the effects of the "body burden" of chemicals has been slow to get recognition (and funding); when Carson was writing, only a handful of scientists and doctors were even thinking about this. It wasn't until 1999 that the Centers for Disease Control (CDC) started a systematic investigation of the accumulation of chemicals in the bodies of Americans. Using medical interviews, physical exams, and samples of serum, blood and urine, the CDC has designed a longitudinal "biomonitoring" program to trace the body burden of a wide range of environmental chemicals (CDC, 2009). Biomonitoring is now a rapidly growing medical subfield.

The findings of several of the most recent biomonitoring studies are shocking, although perhaps Carson herself wouldn't be surprised: more than 90 percent of US residents carry some mixture of pesticide residues in their bodies; the average number of pesticides detected was 13. The 2009 CDC study revealed that body burdens for two of the pesticides studied were three to almost five times beyond the "acceptable range" (CDC, 2009; Pesticide Action Network, 2004).

Disease outcomes

Carson couldn't "prove" a specific correlation between pesticide residues in human bodies and specific health effects. Because of the space/time gap between exposures and outcomes, it was then—and remains today—virtually impossible to "prove" correlations. But she assembles virtually all the evidence then known that pointed strongly in the direction of particular health problems, which include the following.

Nervous system disorders

It was well known, as Carson was writing *Silent Spring*, that most of the pesticides in use could cause damage to the nervous system—sometimes acute and fatal, sometimes delayed and seemingly manageable (things such as memory loss, insomnia, nightmares). Cases of paralysis, long delayed after acute pesticide exposures, were known and validated by researchers. Medical investigations had already established that lindane, then a favored insecticide (and still available today in the United States as a pharmaceutical treatment for lice or scabies), was taken up and stored in large quantities in the brain and liver, and that it had the potential for long-lasting central nervous system effects. Lindane vaporizers were being heavily marketed as Carson was writing—one of the products that Carson rails against at great length.

The organic phosphates, Carson explained, although most notorious for the violent effects of acute poisoning, were also suspected in long-term damage to nerve tissues and seemed to be implicated in the onset of several mental disorders. She argues that, in light of the severe damage the organic phosphates do to the nervous system, it is "perhaps inevitable" (p. 117) that they would be linked to mental disease. She reports on research in Melbourne involving 16 patients with mental disease—from schizophrenia to depression—all of whom had history of prolonged exposure to organic phosphorus insecticides. Three were scientists checking the efficacy of sprays, eight worked in greenhouses, and five were farm workers. All 16 had normal medical histories before they were involved in the spraying. After the spraying, they all suffered confusion, delusions, loss of memory, depression: "a heavy price to pay for the temporary destruction of a few insects, but a price that will continue to be exacted as long as we insist upon using chemicals that strike directly at the nervous system" (pp. 176–178).

Cancers

Carson devotes an entire chapter ("One in Every Four") to contemplating the epidemic of cancer produced by chemical exposures. She starts her exploration with the observation that humans, of all life forms, are the only ones able to *produce* cancer-causing agents. She asserts the indisputable fact that in the modern chemical era, malignancies were increasing at an alarming rate. Careful to provide data where available, Carson paints a grim portrait.

She explores the troubling rise in childhood cancers. Prior to the "pesticide age," cancer in children was considered a medical rarity. And yet, as Carson was writing, more school-age children were dying from cancer than from any other disease: 12 percent, Carson reports, of all deaths in children between the ages of one and fourteen were then caused by cancer. This remains the case today: cancers kill more children under age 14 than any other disease (although accidents cause more deaths in this age group, overall).[11] Carson notes that significant numbers of malignant tumors are discovered clinically in children under the age of five, and even more worrying, that significant numbers of children are born with malignancies.

Carson noted with alarm that with the rise of modern pesticides came significant increases in the incidence of leukemia. Carson provides figures from the National Office of Vital Statistics that tracked a disturbing rise in malignant diseases of the blood and blood-forming tissues. She writes that in 1960, leukemia alone killed more than 12,000 Americans, and almost 25,000 died from all types of blood and lymphatic malignancies (a sharp increase from 17,000 in 1950). "In terms of deaths per 100,000 of population, the increase is from 11.1 in 1950 to 14.1 in 1960" (p. 202). Increases in leukemia were global, and rising at a rate of 4–5 percent a year.

Carson chillingly notes that certain chemicals, reminiscent of radioactive substances such as strontium-90, "have a peculiar affinity" (p. 209) for bone marrow. For example, benzene was a common constituent of insecticides—and is a chemical basis for lindane, the perils of which Carson has already revealed. Carson knew that benzene had long been identified in the medical literature as a cause of leukemia.

But Carson knew that the insidious time-lag between exposure to chemicals and manifestations of cancer meant that much of the medical evidence would be considered to be "circumstantial." Ironically, although the United States was awash in pesticides as Carson was writing *Silent Spring*, not enough time had passed to be able to identify the health effects of the new chlorinated hydrocarbon pesticides. As Carson notes, most malignancies in people develop so slowly that several decades could pass before detectable symptoms emerged. Carson's grave prognostication was that "[t]he full maturing of whatever seeds of malignancy have been sown by these chemicals is yet to come" (p. 201).

And Carson again emphasizes the importance of synergies, and raises the specter of the particular threat of a looming deadly synergy between radiation and pesticides. Human exposures to cancer-causing agents are uncontrolled, often unknown, and they are multiple. Any given individual may be exposed to any given chemical several times over in different contexts and different forms. Carson gives the example of arsenic, which ordinary people encountered ubiquitously in their everyday lives:

> [A]s an air pollutant, a contaminant of water, a pesticide residue on food, in medicines, cosmetics, wood preservatives, or as a coloring agent in paints and inks. It is quite possible that no one of these exposures alone would be sufficient to precipitate malignancy—yet any single supposedly "safe dose" may be enough to tip the scales that are already loaded with other "safe doses."
>
> (p. 211)

Carson also warns us that health damage can be the result of two or more carcinogens acting together. For example, she pointed out that people exposed to liver-damaging DDT were almost certain to *also* be exposed to other liver-damaging hydrocarbons that were, even then, almost ubiquitous in the everyday environment in products such as paint removers, solvents, dry-cleaning fluids, and degreasing agents. Under such circumstances, she asks almost rhetorically, "What then can be a 'safe dose' of DDT?" (p. 211). Cancer, she asserts, often derives not from any single exposure, but from the combined, "complementary" action of two or more chemicals.

> Thus, the herbicides IPC and CIPC may act as initiators in the production of skin tumors, sowing the seeds of malignancy that may be brought into actual being by something else—perhaps a common detergent. There may be interaction, too, between a physical and a chemical agent. Leukemia may occur as a two-step process, the malignant change being initiated by X-radiation, the promoting action being supplied by a chemical, as, for example, urethane. The growing exposure of the population to radiation from various sources, plus the many contacts with a host of chemicals suggest a grave new problem for the modern world.
> (pp. 211–212)

Interestingly enough, Carson doesn't discuss breast cancer anywhere in the book. It is not clear whether this reflects a lack of medical literature on breast cancer at the time she was writing, or a reluctance to enter what could be fraught personal terrain. Nonetheless, she has subsequently become a symbol for contemporary organizing around breast cancer in the environmental movement. In Carson's name and spirit, feminists who have insisted on bridging the women's health/environmental gap—in the 1980s and 1990s, facing an uphill battle within the environmental movement itself—are transforming the state of knowledge about the environmental causes of breast cancer (see also Seager, 2003). National women's groups such as Breast Cancer Action (http://www.bcaction.org/) and the Silent Spring Institute (http://www.silentspring.org/) track medical research, collect community-based information about breast cancer clusters, and through their advocacy they shape the research focus of medical and environmental science.

Largely because of such efforts, the most intense focus of medical investigation of breast cancer these days is the relationship of pesticides to the cancer. Why this particular relationship? Many pesticides mimic estrogen, a known breast cancer risk factor. There is increasing evidence that many synthetic chemicals interfere with our bodies' complex and carefully regulated hormonal system—a phenomenon known as "endocrine disruption." Chemicals disrupt the endocrine system in several ways, including mimicking or blocking chemicals naturally found in the body, altering hormonal levels, and altering the body's ability to produce hormones. Endocrine disruption—of which estrogen mimicry is one example—is linked to dozens of health effects, including low sperm counts, reproductive failures, infertility, and hormonally generated cancers, such as breast and prostate cancer.

Suspected endocrine disrupting chemicals are found in insecticides, herbicides, fumigants, and fungicides that are widely used in agriculture as well as in the home. Other endocrine disruptors are found in industrial chemicals such as detergents, resins, plasticizers, and monomers in many plastics. Exposure to these chemicals occurs through direct contact in the workplace or at home, or through ingestion of contaminated water, food, or air. Studies have found that some of these chemicals leach out of plastics, such as the PVC plastics used to make IV bags. When these plastics, or other materials, are burned (as well as in their production), many unwanted by-products that are endocrine disruptors or suspected endocrine disruptors are released into the air, water, or food. Most endocrine disrupting chemicals are fat-soluble, which means that they don't get rapidly flushed out of the body, but rather are stored in fat.[12]

The publication of an astonishing book in 1996, *Our Stolen Future*, catapulted endocrine disruption into American consciousness and put it on the public health agenda (Colborn et al., 1996). Like *Silent Spring*, *Our Stolen Future* was a "popularized" synthesis of the state-of-the-art scientific understanding of the endocrinal effects of synthetic chemicals. When Carson was writing, "endocrine disruption" was not yet on any medical or scientific agenda. The evidence emerging in the 1950s of DDT's effect on reproduction in birds was one of the first indications of the impact of chemicals on the endocrine system. Carson had her finger on this pulse of the cutting-edge research that would, several decades later, reveal the enormity of the endocrine disruption problem.

The chlorinated hydrocarbon pesticides (DDT, dieldrin, etc.), Carson says, are particularly likely to have both a hormonal as well as an "indirect carcinogenesis" effect—because they damage the liver. The liver acts as the protection against excess accumulation of the sex hormones, helping to sustain the balance between male and female hormones. The liver can't play this role if it's damaged. And in the absence of a well-functioning liver, the estrogens can build up to excessively high levels. She goes on to report on the handful of studies available at that time that provided specific findings of tumor growth when estrogen levels were elevated.

Carson admits that "medical opinion was divided" on what we would now call endocrine disruption, but she warns that it is a "serious" concern that will need further attention—a prophetic entreaty.

Cellular mutation

Carson was deeply interested in the ways that radiation caused cellular mutations, and it was her understanding of the effects of radiation exposure that led her to make the direct comparison with synthetic chemicals. The fact that Carson devoted an entire chapter (Chapter 13, "Through a Narrow Window") to genetics was in itself a remarkable feat of research—and reach—and signaled the importance she accorded to this new field of inquiry. For most readers of *Silent Spring*, "genetics" and "cellular mutagenesis" would be new ground. Before she could make the case about the mutagenic effects of chemicals, Carson had to first educate the public about cell biology—which she did in a remarkable three pages in Chapter 13.

Research on the disruptive effects of *radiation* on cellular-level processes would be familiar to the more science-literate segment of the American public by the late 1950s, largely due to the award of the Nobel Prize in Medicine to Dr. Hermann Muller for his discovery of the multiple-generational effects of mutations caused by radiation. Carson certainly understood the state-of-the-art scientific knowledge about the damage to cells caused by radiation: cells exposed to radiation stopped dividing normally, the structure of chromosomes was damaged, and genes could be deformed, causing next-generation effects. If especially susceptible, cells could be killed outright through exposure to radiation, or could, years later, become malignant.

What Carson does with this information about radiation, though, is extraordinary. Working through the material on genetics and radiation, she takes the leap into the study of the mutagenesis of chemicals. Carson is well ahead of her time when she argues that the parallel between chemicals and radiation "is exact and inescapable." She remarks that laboratory studies had established the fact that a large group of chemicals reproduced radiomimetic (radiation-mimicking) consequences:

> Many chemicals used as pesticides—herbicides as well as insecticides—belong to this group of substances that have the ability to damage the chromosomes, interfere with normal cell division, or cause mutations. These injuries to the genetic material are of a kind that may lead to disease in the individual exposed or they may make their effects felt in future generations.
> (p. 186)

The entire field of cellular study and genetics was so new and unfamiliar that very few scientists could claim expertise. As Carson said, the study of chromosomes was still in its infancy—it was only in 1956 that scientists determined accurately the number of human chromosomes.

Even fewer researchers, when Carson was writing *Silent Spring*, had made the leap that Carson did from studying radiation to research on *chemicals* and genetic mutation. The idea of studying the effect of environmental factors on chromosomes was a radical innovation. "The whole concept of genetic damage by something in the environment," she writes, "is relatively new, and is little understood except by the geneticists, whose advice is too seldom sought" (p. 189).

Carson uncovered one important research effort, which she said was the first study of chemical mutagenic effects. In the 1940s, Charlotte Auerbach and William Robson at the University of Edinburgh experimented with mustard gas on fruit flies—the same organisms Muller had used for his radiation studies. They found that the gas produced permanent chromosome abnormalities that were indistinguishable from those induced by radiation. Carson reported on the scattering of other research on chemicals and cellular mutations, but there was little to go on. There was some evidence that the popular herbicide, 2,4-D, produced chromosomal changes in plants and retarded cell division, but, when Carson was writing, there had been no comprehensive study aimed at testing the mutagenic effects of pesticides—as there would not be for two more decades.

In the midst of the atomic age, the implications of work on cellular mutations were enormous. Muller's work was under scrutiny and challenge, and his ideas were denounced and resisted by many. Carson knew that to venture into the world of chemical mutagenesis would be even more controversial: "The fact that chemicals may play a role similar to radiation has scarcely dawned on the public mind, nor on the minds of most medical or scientific workers" (p. 190).

Carson was determined to rouse scientific and public attention to this issue. Throughout *Silent Spring*, Carson typically refrained from using alarmist language, but on the issue of mutagenesis she thought there was not enough alarm: "[G]enetic deterioration through man-made agents is the menace of our time, 'the last and greatest danger to our civilization'" (p. 186), she proclaimed. She ended the chapter with a denunciation:

> We can, if we wish, reduce this threat to our genetic heritage, a possession that has come down to us through some two billion years of evolution and selection of living protoplasm, a possession that is ours for the moment only, until we must pass it on to generations to come. We are doing little now to preserve its integrity. Although chemical manufacturers are required by law to test their materials for toxicity, they are not required to make the tests that would reliably demonstrate genetic effect, and they do not do so.
>
> (p. 194)

For further discussion/exploration

- Is it possible to have a large-scale commercial agricultural system based on zero-level tolerance for pesticide residues on foods?

- Identify five of your own favorite foods and see what you can find out about their pesticide residue profiles.

- Has a recent "food scare" caught your attention? What roles have been played in addressing the problem by state and federal government agencies? Have they been in agreement about the nature of the problem?

- Carson was concerned that news about her own cancer might have fueled accusations by critics that she was not able to be objective or unbiased in her critique of pesticides. Do you think that would have been the case? Would it be the case today?

- Why do you think Carson doesn't mention breast cancer in the entire book?

- Choose one popular lawn-care pesticide product and examine how it is marketed. What are the gender, race, and class images associated with the product?

- What pesticide products have been withdrawn from the market, and why?

- What is a "safe level of use," and how do we know?

5

Alternatives

Having painted a depressing portrait of the many ways in which humans were threatening and degrading all life, did Carson see any alternative? What would Carson do differently? What would she have *us* do?

Passion, wonder, and beauty

Although it may seem hard to detect, Carson was an optimist. Carson saw no reason that we should create—or accept—life with "only its head out of water, inches above the limits of toleration of the corruption of its own environment". She loved life. She loved the birds, she felt kinship with the sea, she loved the woods. She thought that ecosystems were wondrous, the web of interconnected life marvelous, the ebb and flow of life filled with beauty. The urgency that compelled her to warn us about the impending danger we were bringing upon ourselves was driven by a passion for the planet.

And it was through passion, wonder, and beauty that she saw one path forward. Carson was convinced that we would not allow ourselves to destroy this wondrous planet if we allowed ourselves to see its wondrousness. "I believe that the more clearly we can focus our attention on the wonders and realities of the universe about us, the less taste we shall have for destruction," she told an audience of women journalists in 1954 (Carson, 1998b, p. 163).

"Wonder" was a trait she felt had been suppressed by science and by the privileging of science as the primary lens through which to comprehend the world. Carson was not anti-science—far from it—and, indeed, she witnessed the many ways in which science *could* reveal the wonders and beauty of nature, and she devoted her own life as a scientist towards that goal. But she also felt that a clinical investigation of the laws of nature was an enterprise quite different from reveling in the beauty and marvel of the world. "Most of us walk unseeing through the world," she writes in *Silent Spring*, "unaware alike of its beauties, its wonders, and the strange and sometimes terrible intensity of the lives that are being lived about us" (p. 220).

Although Carson wrote *Silent Spring* with a polemical agenda in mind, and as a very different book than her previous three, the naturewriter in her didn't disappear. She not only talks about beauty, she *shows* us the beauty of the nature she fears will disappear. *Silent Spring* has breathtaking passages where Carson's writing soars to put beauty before us in a tangible way.

Carson also talked about a notion related to beauty and wonder, that of humility—or, rather, our loss of humility. In the hustle and bustle of contemporary life, Carson says, it is easy to forget that human life is entirely dependent on plants—for photosynthesis, for harnessing solar energy, and, of course, for food.

> The earth's vegetation is part of a web of life in which there are intimate and essential relations between plants and the earth, between plants and other plants, between plants and animals. Sometimes we have no choice but to disturb these relationships, but we should do so thoughtfully, with full awareness that what we do may have consequences remote in time and place. But no such humility marks the booming "weed killer" business of the present day, in which soaring sales and expanding uses mark the production of plant-killing chemicals.
>
> (p. 64)

And in the penultimate paragraph of *Silent Spring*, she laments that a chemical barrage has been hurled against the fabric of life:

> A fabric on the one hand delicate and destructible, on the other miraculously tough and resilient, and capable of striking back in

unexpected ways. These extraordinary capacities of life have been ignored by the practitioners of chemical control who have brought to their task no "high-minded orientation," no humility before the vast forces with which they tamper.

(p. 261)

"Humility" often has religious overtones, but Carson's invocation is not a religious one. She is speaking to the rash overconfidence of humans who act as though they can remove themselves from the inescapable truth that humans are part of nature. Humility was embedded in her ecological message that we are all part of nature, and that our efforts to put ourselves outside of natural cycles (or, more likely, above them) will backfire. Humans are not better than, bigger than, stronger than, or outside of nature, Carson would say, and it is when we lose sight of that truth that we get ourselves into trouble.

It was "wonder" that brought Carson to nature; it was wonder that kept her gaze focused there. In 1956, Carson wrote an essay, "Help Your Child to Wonder," published in *Woman's Home Companion*. She had intended to expand this into a book—a project that she never completed. The book, *The Sense of Wonder*, was published posthumously in 1965. *The Sense of Wonder* is Carson's ode to the beauty of nature. Carson felt that adulthood often dimmed the sense of wonder that came to children easily: "It is our misfortune that for most of us, that clear-eyed vision, that true instinct for what is beautiful and awe-inspiring, is dimmed and even lost before we reach adulthood . . . a sense of wonder . . . is an unfailing antidote against the boredom and disenchantments of later years, the sterile preoccupation with things that are artificial, the alienation from our sources of strength . . . it is not half so important to *know as to feel*" (Carson, 1998a, pp. 54–56).

The "misfortune" of our loss of wonder and our loss of the capacity to apprehend beauty in nature is a theme that bookends *Silent Spring*. Carson uses the word "misfortune" sparingly, only twice in *Silent Spring*—once at the beginning, and once at the very end. Carson concludes her opening fable of the town overcome by silence by noting that the town does not really exist, but that it has a thousand counterparts across America:

> I know of no community that has experienced all the misfortunes I describe. Yet every one of these disasters has actually happened somewhere ... A grim specter has crept upon us almost unnoticed, and this imagined tragedy may easily become a stark reality we all shall know.
>
> (pp. 14–15)

And the very last sentence of the book ends with "misfortune":

> It is our alarming misfortune that so primitive a science has armed itself with the most modern and terrible weapons, and that in turning them against the insects it has also turned them against the earth.
>
> (p. 262)

With its wistful sadness, "misfortune" is a word that is both an unmistakable admonishment, used as Carson does, and yet holds out a kernel of redemptive possibility. And that *is* the tension underlying *Silent Spring*—the message that we have really screwed up, but that we can do better.

Pragmatic alternatives

Invoking Robert Frost's two roads, Carson writes:

> The road we have long been traveling is deceptively easy, a smooth superhighway on which we progress with great speed, but at its end lies disaster. The other fork of the road—the one "less traveled by"—offers our last, our only chance to reach a destination that assures the preservation of our earth.
>
> (p. 244)

Carson was not a romantic idealist. She knew that wonder and beauty would not, alone, catalyze the changes in human behavior that were needed. As a pragmatic matter of science and biology, Carson was certain that there were specific alternatives to the indiscriminate saturation of the environment with pesticides. She devoted her last chapter (Chapter 17, "The Other Road") to an exploration of those alternatives.

Natural controls

Carson's research brought her into contact with cutting-edge investigation of biological controls that could be used to contain or kill unwanted insects and plants. She said, after all, this was how a natural balance was maintained. The world of insects, she asserted, is one held in natural balance. Populations of insects fluctuate with food supply, changing weather and climate conditions, and the presence of competing or predatory species; it is, as often as not, insects that keep other insects in check. One of the significant problems with chemical control is that the chemicals kill all insects indiscriminately—"friends" and "enemies" alike. If humans are not going to just leave nature alone, if humans are going to intervene to shape outcomes in the natural world, then Carson says we should be clever enough to intervene by deploying the tools of nature.

She offers dozens of examples of natural and biological controls that had been proven effective, among them:

- introducing natural disease or bacteria to control unwanted insect populations, such as using milky spore disease to control Japanese beetles (pp. 93–95);
- releasing sterilized insects to infiltrate the natural population of the "nuisance" species, thus effecting population reductions, such as proven successes with eradicating the screw-worm fly (pp. 246–247);
- manipulating insect pheromones to deter or deflect reproduction attraction, as had been demonstrated with gypsy moths (pp. 252–253);
- controlling unwanted plants by introducing plant-specific insects that eat the plants, as with the Klamath weed in the American west (pp. 80–81);
- replacing the toxic pesticides (especially the chlorinated hydrocarbons) with naturally derived pesticides such as pyrethrins or rotenone, synthesized from plants (p. 166).

Humans, she said, should be smart enough to work *with* nature, not only against it. Carson points to the evidence that biological controls have had spectacular successes in curbing unwanted vegetation and insects. Using "nature herself" (p. 80), she says, will solve problems in the most successful way.

Carson understands that introducing biological controls often means introducing new organisms into an ecosystem—and that no matter how targeted the introduction, this might have unintended consequences. She doesn't address this directly in *Silent Spring*, but her position would most likely be that the unintended consequences of biological controls would not be—*could* not be—as devastating as the systemic poisoning of the world with pesticides.

In her advocacy for "natural controls" of agricultural pests, Carson is previewing the work that has led to an agricultural system now known as "integrated pest management" (IPM)—which, when Carson was writing, was in its nascent days. The US EPA, which heavily promotes IPM, describes it as a set of "common-sense," environmentally sensitive practices. Farmers who practice IPM don't use pesticides at the first sign of an insect—although, eventually, this may be part of the solution to an agricultural pest infestation. Rather, the EPA describes these steps as follows:[1]

> IPM is not a single pest control method but, rather, a series of pest management evaluations, decisions and controls. In practicing IPM, growers who are aware of the potential for pest infestation follow a four-tiered approach. The four steps include:
>
> - **Set Action Thresholds:** Before taking any pest control action, IPM first sets an action threshold, a point at which pest populations or environmental conditions indicate that pest control action must be taken. Sighting a single pest does not always mean control is needed. The level at which pests will either become an economic threat is critical to guide future pest control decisions.
>
> - **Monitor and Identify Pests:** Not all insects, weeds, and other living organisms require control. Many organisms are innocuous, and some are even beneficial. IPM programs work to monitor for pests and identify them accurately, so

that appropriate control decisions can be made in conjunction with action thresholds. This monitoring and identification removes the possibility that pesticides will be used when they are not really needed or that the wrong kind of pesticide will be used.

- **Prevention:** As a first line of pest control, IPM programs work to manage the crop, lawn, or indoor space to prevent pests from becoming a threat. In an agricultural crop, this may mean using cultural methods, such as rotating between different crops, selecting pest-resistant varieties, and planting pest-free rootstock. These control methods can be very effective and cost-efficient and present little to no risk to people or the environment.

- **Control:** Once monitoring, identification, and action thresholds indicate that pest control is required, and preventive methods are no longer effective or available, IPM programs then evaluate the proper control method both for effectiveness and risk. Effective, less risky pest controls are chosen first, including highly targeted chemicals, such as pheromones to disrupt pest mating, or mechanical control, such as trapping or weeding. If further monitoring, identifications and action thresholds indicate that less risky controls are not working, then additional pest control methods would be employed, such as targeted spraying of pesticides. Broadcast spraying of non-specific pesticides is a last resort.

Selective spraying

As established earlier, Carson was not entirely opposed to the use of pesticides. She understood that pesticides might be, under some circumstances, warranted. What she was ferociously opposed to was the irresponsible and wanton spraying of pesticides.

The alternative? *Selective* spraying, of course. The technique of applying poisons only to the plants one is trying to get rid of is, to Carson, entirely sensible. This technique, she argued, was especially suited for eliminating "weeds" on highway roadsides or utility rights of way. She gives several examples of successful selective spraying, mentioning particularly the work in developing the technique by a scientist at the American Museum of Natural History. Carson points out that selective spraying was less costly, more efficient, and immeasurably less toxic. Selective spraying reduces dramatically the quantity and frequency of chemical applications, in turn reducing most of the "collateral" damage to other plants and to wildlife. And yet, selective spraying, as Carson was writing, had only been adopted in a few places:

> For the most part, entrenched custom dies hard and blanket spraying continues to thrive, to exact its heavy annual costs from the taxpayer, and to inflict its damage on the ecological web of life. It thrives, surely, only because the facts are not known.
>
> (p. 75)

In this passage, we see also Carson's hope that when citizens *know* more, they will act differently—or will insist that their government agencies and municipal governments do so. But to Carson, the problem of expanding the knowledge base wasn't just one of expanding the circle of formal education about science and ecosystems and health impacts of certain chemicals. Carson was particularly enthusiastic about knowledge from the bottom up—what we might now call "citizen science."

Citizen science

Carson had enormous respect for the dedicated amateur. She knew that "nature appreciation"—whether backyard bird-feeding, gardening, birdwatching, mushroom-collecting, hiking, even fishing—absorbed millions of Americans. Their regular ongoing contact with nature, their observations of the natural world, often positioned these nature-engaged ordinary citizens to be the most reliable narrators of changes or disruptions to the environment. Carson became actively engaged with the fight against pesticides in 1957 and 1958, when Olga Huckins, a writer and editor, contacted her about the devastation from spraying in her backyard sanctuary in Duxbury, Massachusetts. The year before, a "group of Long Island citizens" (p. 144), so named in Carson's account even though they included several highly-placed lawyers and professionals, pressed a lawsuit against spraying and took it all the way to the Supreme Court; they lost the case but put pesticide spraying on the national map. Carson was discouraged that the Long Island group lost the court battle, but she credited their fight with putting pesticides on the public agenda. The Long Island case, she says, was the wake-up call for most middle-class Americans who could see in that battle their own concerns about private property rights and the right to control one's own health choices.

In describing the devastation of spraying to prevent Dutch elm disease in Wisconsin, Carson reports on the work of scientist naturalists *and* the letters from citizens that sparked outrage. Carson says that anywhere there has been spraying, letters-from-readers columns of the local newspapers are full of angry, indignant, and sad letters from citizens who, in Carson's view, display a greater knowledge of the dangers of spraying than the officials who are in charge:

> "I am dreading the days to come soon now when many beautiful birds will be dying in our back yard," wrote a Milwaukee woman. "This is a pitiful, heartbreaking experience . . . It is, moreover, frustrating and exasperating, for it evidently does not serve the purpose this slaughter was intended to serve . . . Taking a long look, can you save trees without also saving birds? Do they not, in the economy of nature, save each other?"
>
> (pp. 106–107)

Carson sprinkles *Silent Spring* with examples of the occasions on which it is citizens who first noticed and first objected to the devastation of pesticides. In Carson's view, the experts often followed in their wake, "confirming" what the amateur observers already knew.

Citizen science is now a legitimate dimension of scientific inquiry.[2] As a "movement," citizen science coalesced in the early 1970s with the formation of groups such as "Science for the People," dedicated initially to exposing the ways science was co-opted to support the US war in Vietnam. Now, "citizen scientists" (a term coined in the 1990s) count birds every December in an organized nationwide census; community groups track cancer clusters; "ordinary housewives" measure pollution in their neighborhood;

others pay to be assistants on "Earthwatch" expeditions; amateur astronomers count asteroids; there are waiting lists for turtle-nesting protection squads. "Crowdsourcing" and Internet technologies have accelerated the opportunities for everyday encounters with and participation in the conduct of science. We've come a long way from Carson's "appreciation of" the role of the amateur observer and activist, but she was ahead of her time even with that appreciation.

Scientific uncertainty

In *Silent Spring*, Carson keeps drawing our attention to how much we don't know about pesticides—their persistence, their synergistic and cumulative effects, their transport and spread through ecosystems and across species, their health effects. At several junctures in the book, she reminds her readers that we have launched ourselves, unwittingly, into a real-time experiment. She means this with reference to specific pesticide programs for which the long-term outcome was entirely uncertain (or, even, unquestioned), but she also means this as a meta-theme: we humans are running full tilt forward into a yawning unknown, spray-gun in hand. As she says repeatedly throughout *Silent Spring* in various ways, no one can tell what the ultimate costs and consequences will be. Recently, scholars tallied Carson's use of terminology that framed the rhetorical ways in which she foregrounded uncertainty in *Silent Spring*: they found 14 uses of "we do not know"; seven uses of "potential for harm"; six uses of "little understood"; four uses of "more research is needed"; and two uses of "lack of consensus" (Walker and Walsh, 2012, pp. 14–15).

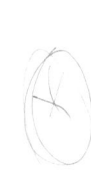

The position of scientific uncertainty—what we collectively "do" with it—is a high-stakes public policy struggle, nowhere more intense than in the environmental field. Particularly in the context of American public policy, uncertainty is conventionally used to support the *status quo* and the presumption that continued forward movement is the most appropriate (lowest cost) response: if we don't *know for sure* that CO_2 emissions are producing climate change, then there's no reason to burden ourselves with regulations against CO_2 emissions until we do know for sure, given the economic disruptions that reductions or a ban would cause; if we don't *know* that exposure to a particular chemical or drug causes breast cancer, then the economic penalty of ceasing production is not warranted.

In many recent policy controversies in the United States, industry representatives or conservatives who deny the legitimacy of science leverage scientific uncertainty into a rationale to delay or block regulatory action (see Michaels, 2008; Oreskes and Conway, 2010; Walker and Walsh, 2012). The "winning party" in debates that pivot around uncertainty is the one who can supply the most compelling portrait of possible outcomes (Walker and Walsh, 2012, p. 7). Uncertainty is often manipulated to sway action—or lack of action—in the favor of powerful interests. Uncertainty can also be created, or exaggerated.

A recent book, *Merchants of Doubt* (Oreskes and Conway, 2010), chronicles the ways in which certain industries, from tobacco to fossil fuels, not only exploit "doubt" as an industrial strategy—to deflect legislation, to confuse the public and regulators, and to maintain "business as usual"—but create it. Climate change denial, for example, is today a well-funded enterprise. In the United States there are several think tanks devoted entirely to sowing seeds of doubt about the certainty that human-induced climate change is underway. If the public is confused about climate change, it has been *made* confused. As Oreskes and Conway establish, often it is the *same* paid scientists who are called on to be the expert doubters across a range of issues:

> In case after case . . . a handful of scientists joined forces with think tanks and private corporations to challenge scientific evidence on a host of contemporary issues. In the early years, much of the money came from the tobacco industry; in later years it came from foundations, think tanks, and the fossil fuel industry. They claimed the link between smoking and cancer remained unproven. They insisted that scientists were mistaken about the risks and limitations of SDI [Reagan's "Star Wars" Strategic Defense Initiative]. They argued that acid rain was caused by volcanoes, and so was the ozone hole . . . they dismissed the reality of global warming. First they claimed there was none, then

they claimed it was just natural variation, and then they claimed that even if it was happening and it was our fault, it didn't matter because we could just adapt to it.

(Oreskes and Conway, 2010, pp. 6–7)

Carson, too, wrestled with the manufacturing of false consent about pesticides, and the collusion of some scientists with the chemical industry to lull the public into believing that the risks of pesticides were "uncertain" and the benefits unassailably certain. Carson was exposing two kinds of uncertainty about pesticides: that of ignorance (often willful—not enough time has been taken, not enough money has been spent, too much secrecy has been built into the system to be able to find or share knowledge); and that based on risk assessment (outcomes are unclear, multiple outcomes are possible, some outcomes may be beneficial, others harmful).

Carson had no patience with willful ignorance. And much ignorance she saw as willful. She was dismayed by managers in agencies and politicians in government who intentionally underfunded programs that were designed to measure the effects of pesticides on health and environment, or to protect the public from industrial harm; as she poignantly pointed out, in most pesticide programs there was enough funding to keep the chemicals flowing, scarcely any for investigating the consequences. She was disdainful of policies that were made in collusion with industry agents who would directly profit from one policy outcome over another. And she was alarmed by the presumption that one could "act now, worry later." In her Preface to the 1961 reissue of *The Sea Around Us,* Carson asserted, with reference to radioactive waste dumping into the oceans, that technology was outpacing knowledge, and that "to dispose first and investigate later is an invitation to disaster" (cited in Lear, 2009, p. 373). In a 1963, post-*Silent Spring* lecture, Carson quoted Barry Commoner in pointing out that we often defer an inquiry into "impacts" until it is far too late:

> The lack of foresight [about introducing harmful substances into the environment] is one of the most serious complications . . . we seldom if ever evaluate the risks associated with a new technological program before it is put into effect. We wait until the

process has become embedded in a vast economic and political commitment, and then it is virtually impossible to alter.

(1998b, p. 232)

But even were we to be more foresightful—as Carson would argue we *must* be—the other kind of uncertainty is not necessarily assuaged: we may "look before we leap," but when we look, there may be contradictory evidence, or, as in the case of pesticides and human health, often the evidence will only emerge over a long time horizon.

What then? Carson answers firmly:

And if . . . we have concluded that we are being asked to take senseless and frightening risks, then we should no longer accept the counsel of those who tell us that we must fill our world with poisonous chemicals; we should look about and see what other course is open to us.

(p. 244)

In this particular context, Carson's "other course" was her interest in biological and natural controls. But her warning that too much was at stake to take "senseless and frightening risks" was one of the overarching themes through *Silent Spring*. What Carson was advocating anticipates what we now call the "precautionary principle"—once again, she was remarkably ahead of her time.

Although there are many "common-sense" precursors to the precautionary principle (including folk aphorisms such as "look before you leap," or "better safe than sorry"), the formal elaboration of an environmental precautionary principle didn't cohere until 1998 at the Wingspread Conference on the Precautionary Principle.[3] Thirty-five scientists, environmentalists, academics, and public intellectuals gathered at the Wingspread conference center in Wisconsin to give shape to the idea that if a harm is predicted but not proven, caution is often warranted—including "doing nothing" (i.e., *not* releasing the chemical, *not* allowing a development to go forward). The consensus prelude to the statement of principles includes these observations:

- We believe existing environmental regulations and other decisions, particularly those based on risk assessment, have failed to protect adequately human health and the environment—the larger system of which humans are but a part.

- We believe there is compelling evidence that damage to humans and the worldwide environment is of such magnitude and seriousness that new principles for conducting human activities are necessary.

- While we realize that human activities may involve hazards, people must proceed more carefully than has been the case in recent history. Corporations, government entities, organizations, communities, scientists and other individuals must adopt a precautionary approach to all human endeavors.

Following from this, the key elements of the principles of precaution include these:

- When an activity raises threats of harm to human health or the environment, precautionary measures should be taken *even if some cause and effect relationships are not fully established scientifically.*

- In this context the proponent of an activity, rather than the public, should bear the burden of proof.

- The process of applying the precautionary principle must be open, informed and democratic and must include potentially affected parties.

- Applying the precautionary principle must also involve an examination of the full range of alternatives, including no action.

This points to a radical realignment of social—and industrial—priorities. It's also very hard to enact; one can immediately imagine a dozen scenarios in which waiting/doing nothing/looking for alternatives seems balky, expensive, impractical. But employing precautionary principles is perhaps considerably less challenging (and in the long run, healthier, in every sense of the word) than rushing forward just because, as Carson would say, we already feel invested in that course of action. The challenge of converting precautionary principles into real-world policy has been taken up by the European Union which, as of 2000, is committed to enacting the environmental Precautionary Principle:

> [European] Union policy on the environment shall aim at a high level of protection taking into account the diversity of situations in the various regions of the Union. It shall be based on the precautionary principle and on the principles that preventive action should be taken, that environmental damage should as a priority be rectified at source and that the polluter should pay.
>
> (Article 191, Lisbon Treaty, 2000)

Carson would have been at Wingspread. She would have signed the statement of principles. She would have written the principles—in some ways, she had already started to.

For further discussion/exploration

- I have identified some lyrical passages from *Silent Spring*, but there are many others. Find an example or two of what you think are her most poetic or "beauty-invoking" passages and discuss the effect such passages have on you as a reader. Do you think Carson strikes an effective balance between the "science" in her book and the "nature appreciation"?

- *Silent Spring* can be seen as an extended critique of human interference with nature, and "experiments" with nature that have gone terribly wrong—or are quite likely to in the future. And yet many of Carson's alternatives to pesticides involve the introduction of new species, or the biological manipulation of others. To what extent do you think this is a contradiction? Does Carson herself explore or discuss the environmental implications of her "alternatives"?

- Are there other governments or jurisdictions that have formally adopted "precautionary principles"?

- What do you think are the biggest problems in "enacting" environmental precautionary principles?

- Have you ever participated as a community member in a science project? What are the limits of "ordinary citizens" participating in science (assuming those individuals are not formally trained in any of the sciences)? What are the benefits—to the participants, to the science enterprise?

6

Responses to *Silent Spring*

In his 1972 biography of Carson, Paul Brooks, her long-time friend and editor at Houghton Mifflin, summarized *Silent Spring* as "one of those rare books that change the course of history—not through incitement to war or violent revolution, but by altering the direction of man's thinking" (Brooks, 1972, p. 227). It is hard to imagine today's environmental movement—and discourse—without the reference baseline (whether in praise or criticism) of *Silent Spring*.

A vast literature assesses and describes the responses to *Silent Spring*. I point to some of this literature in "Sources for further reading and research," below. Literally hundreds of articles and dozens of books tell the story of *Silent Spring*'s reception. Rather than repeat a well-told story here, my goal in this chapter is to briefly outline the nature of the responses and bring it up to date.

A book like no other

The New Yorker release, and then the book itself, set off a tidal wave of activity. Carson was in considerable demand. In advance of *The New Yorker* release, Carson had been active on the lecture circuit. She was quite ill by the time *Silent Spring* was released, and she wanted to reduce the hectic schedule she had been keeping, but the demand for the author was high. As Linda Lear notes:

> Marie Rodell was swamped with requests for interviews and articles . . . The London *Sunday Times* wanted an interview, Richard Arlett of NBC called to ask if Carson would be interviewed on the

Today show by Hugh Downs, National EducationalTV wanted to film a segment on *Silent Spring*, and Caedmon Records wanted to discuss a record contract of Carson reading from her sea books. Rodell gave a polite no to most of these on Carson's behalf.
(Lear, 2009, p. 415)

The promotion machinery for the book was in high gear: the Consumer's Union ordered a special 40,000 copy print-run of the book to distribute to their members; *Reader's Digest* inquired about a condensation; the Book of the Month Club designated *Silent Spring* as their October 1962 featured book, with a first printing of 150,000 copies; the book was nominated for the 1963 National Book Award, (but lost out to Leon Edel's tome on Henry James); Congressman John Lindsay read into the *Congressional Record* several paragraphs of *Silent Spring*; the Audubon Society published lengthy excerpts from the book in its magazine; *CBS Reports* aired a special TV show on *Silent Spring* watched by an estimated audience of 10–15 million people, amounting to, as Linda Lear says, "virtually another special printing of *Silent Spring*" (Lear, 2009, p. 450). Carson became a household name.

And not just in the United States. Translations were published in German in 1962; in French, Swedish, Danish, Dutch, Finnish, and Italian in 1963; in Spanish, Portuguese, and Japanese in 1964; as well as in Icelandic in 1965 and Norwegian in 1966. Abridged selections also appeared on the pages of popular periodicals. Hundreds of thousands who never picked up the book could read Carson's words on the pages of the popular French magazine *Paris-Match* and the regional newspaper *La Dépêche du Midi*, the Italian journal *L'Europeo*, the Dutch weekly newspaper *Elseviers Weekblad*, the Swedish magazine *Vi*, or *Helsingin Sanomat*, the largest Finnish newspaper. Dozens of reviews appeared in every major Western European nation as well as in Hungary and Yugoslavia.[1]

The US government—or, rather, parts of it—acted with alacrity. Disturbed by the excerpts of *Silent Spring* in *The New Yorker*, President Kennedy instructed the President's Science Advisory Committee (PSAC) to investigate Carson's claims. In May 1963, the PSAC released its report. Carson and most of the press regarded the PSAC report as a vindication of *Silent Spring* and of Carson's grasp of the science of pesticides, which itself had come under considerable scrutiny. It was more than just a vindication. Among its many detailed findings, the PSAC confirmed that while pesticide use brought considerable benefits in terms of control of disease and in increasing food production, it also carried considerable risks, including:[2] wide dispersal of pesticides from points of application; pesticide residues routinely found on food items; extreme toxicity and high rates of mortality to non-target organisms; threats to human health, about which the medical community was generally unaware and ill-equipped to handle; astonishingly high rates of use of agricultural pesticides, insecticides, and home-based pesticides that meant that 1 out of every 12 acres of the entire land mass of the United States had been treated with pesticides (as of their writing in 1963); long-term persistence trails from pesticide use that lasted, in many instances, for several years; dangers from low-level, chronic exposure to pesticides that were even more threatening than acute exposures; synergistic effects that were likely to be extremely dangerous, but were largely unknown; and that the current regulatory system was inadequate to the task of protecting safety. The PSAC recommended that investigation into and government support of non-pesticide, biological controls of agricultural pests should be fast-tracked and considerably expanded. The Panel concluded that:

> Public literature and the experiences of Panel members indicate that, until the publication of "Silent Spring" by Rachel Carson, people were generally unaware of the toxicity of pesticides. The government should present this information to the public in a way that will make it aware of the dangers while recognizing the value of pesticides.

Congressional hearings on environmental hazards, including federal regulation of pesticides, were convened by Connecticut Senator Ribicoff; his hearings, at which Carson was a star witness, started the day after the PSAC released its report. Carson's appearances at Ribicoff's hearings, and before another Congressional meeting two days later, were among her last public appearances.

In the wake of *Silent Spring*, Congress revised the regulation of chemicals, although the process was slow and balky. The Nixon administration established the EPA in 1970, and gave it wide-ranging authority over chemicals. Important legislative revisions to the Federal Insecticide, Fungicide, and Rodenticide Act (FIFRA) in 1972, transferred pesticide regulation authority to the EPA (from the Department of Agriculture) and mandated that the EPA emphasize protection of the environment and public health in exercising its scientific and regulatory authority. That same year, following several lawsuits, the EPA banned DDT for use in the United States (though not for export); eventually, the EPA banned or severely restricted five other compounds Carson featured in *Silent Spring*—chlordane (1988), heptachlor (1988), dieldrin (1974), aldrin (1974), and endrin (1986).[3]

The USDA, the government agency that had the greatest stakes in pesticides and that was the most severely critiqued by Carson, seemed remarkably unprepared for the political fallout from *Silent Spring* (Lear, 1992). With public and political scrutiny of the USDA and its research arm, the Agricultural Research Service (ARS), whipped up by Carson's book, the agency seemed caught by surprise and almost immediately struck a defensive posture. With the first two *New Yorker* articles published, the ARS director wrote to Agricultural Secretary Orville Freeman that Carson's "sweeping attack will undermine the public's confidence in the food supplied and safeguarded by state and federal agencies and ought not to be dismissed lightly" (cited in Lear, 1992, p. 161). Realizing they couldn't "dismiss" *Silent Spring*, the agency didn't have a strategy: they didn't know whether to attack Carson's findings, whether to emphasize the benefits that pesticides offer, or whether to strike a conciliatory middle-ground note with an agreement that "more research" would be welcome. In August 1962, after *The New Yorker* installments were out, but before the book was, the USDA released its official response:

> Miss Carson presents a lucid description of the real and potential dangers of misusing chemical pesticides. These are poisonous compounds and, if used improperly, can be dangerous. The [*New Yorker*] articles serve to alert people to this danger. They also emphasize the need for greater public support of efforts to develop more effective biological and non-chemical pest control techniques, to develop more sophisticated chemicals that will affect only one or two species of pests, and to intensify research on the effect of

pesticides on people and animals. She expresses the concern of many people about the effect of chemical pesticides on birds, animals and people. We are fully aware of, and share, this concern.
(cited in Lear, 1993, p. 164)

Despite this conciliatory note, behind the scenes the USDA was providing indirect assistance to the attacks against Carson mounted by the agricultural chemical industry and industrial groups such as the National Pest Control Association.

The chemical industry, especially pesticide manufacturers, was apoplectic about *Silent Spring*—and about Carson herself. Her critics did everything they could to battle back against Carson's arguments. They realized that Carson was not just attacking particular pesticides or practices—they "got it" that she had challenged the design and intent of much of the reigning paradigm of pest control. They understood that Carson's critique was an attack on the entire model of chemical-based insect control. Carson was also challenging the value system that supported the premise of "progress through pesticides."

They didn't want to take on the values debate directly, so industry first focused on the science behind Carson's analysis. They coordinated press conferences and statements from a steady parade of scientists who refuted her claims. Many of these scientists, genuinely believing that their work benefited farmers and helped to feed a growing world, were shocked by the way Carson portrayed them in the sinister context of profit-driven corporations and complicit government and educational institutions. Industry critics challenged her scientific accuracy and acumen, piece by piece; Carson pushed back, supported by a phalanx of other scientists who validated her work. When the PSAC report came out in 1963 essentially endorsing Carson's findings, the line-by-line science debate abated. But by then, the chemical industry had consolidated another line of attack.

They took the tack of providing counter evidence of the good done by pesticides. One of their major arguments was that, without pesticides, agriculture would collapse and pests and pestilence would run amok. Monsanto published a brochure in October 1962 parodying Carson's opening fable of the silent town called "The Desolate Year," dramatizing the poverty and disease of a world without pesticides; 5,000 copies were sent out to editors and book reviewers.[4] Carson's attitude toward pesticides, a review in *Chemical and Engineering News* noted, would mean "disease, epidemics, starvation, misery and suffering incomparable and intolerable to modern man" (Darby, 1962, p. 60). This theme has recently been revived, as we will see below.

Carson herself was as much the subject of attacks as her book. Carson was a threat to her detractors not merely because of her message about pesticides, but because she was a woman, an independent scholar whose sex and lack of institutional ties placed her outside the nexus of production and application of conventional scientific knowledge (Smith, 2001, p. 734). Invoking a familiar Cold War trope, her loyalty as an American was questioned. Ezra Taft Benson, former Agriculture Secretary, privately suggested to former President Dwight Eisenhower that Carson was "probably a communist." A letter to the editor of *The New Yorker* echoed a similar theme:

> Miss Rachel Carson's reference to the selfishness of insecticide manufacturers probably reflects her Communist sympathies, like a lot of our writers these days. We can live without birds and animals, but, as the current market slump shows, we cannot live without business. As for insects, isn't it just like a woman to be scared to death of a few little bugs! As long as we have the H-bomb everything will be O.K.
>
> (cited in Stoll, 2012)

Sexism knew no bounds. Gender was used to denigrate Carson and her science, and the gender-hazing she endured was clearly a tactic by critics to shape the debate over pesticides according to the rules of industrial capitalism—which identified itself with a masculine norm. Carson's writing, combining "caring" with science, was considered to be well beyond the male pale.

Her "love" of nature was seen as evidence of an unserious author. Many male critics castigated her as a "bird and bunny lover." In one remarkable all-in-one critique, the author called her "part of the vociferous, misinformed group of nature balancing, organic gardening, bird loving, unreasonable citizenry" (cited in Trost, 1984, p. 68).

She was portrayed, especially, as a hysterical female who knew little about the ways of the world.[5] A lengthy 1962 review in *Time* magazine (titled, tellingly, "Pesticides: The Price for Progress"), accused her of being emotionally overwrought: "Many scientists sympathize with Miss Carson's love of wildlife, and even with her mystical attachment to the balance of nature. But they fear that her emotional and inaccurate outburst in Silent Spring may do harm by alarming the nontechnical public, while doing no good for the things that she loves" (cited in Lear, 2009, p. 430). The *Time* review went on to accuse Carson of "taking up her pen in anger and alarm" (cited in Trost, 1984, p. 68). One now well-cited review in *Chemical and Engineering News* by a medical doctor, William Darby, noted that "It is doubtful that many readers can bear to wade through its high-pitched sequences of anxieties" (Darby, 1962, p. 61). The *National Review* called the book "simply a long emotional attack" and invoked the need for "rational" and "scientific" approaches in place of Carson's screed (cited in Smith, 2001, p. 741). The vilification of Carson invoked notions of the conduct of "good science" that should be "rational" and "unemotional"; Francis Bacon would be pleased.

Much of the story of Carson and her critics echoes with strains of the triumph of Baconian modern (male) science over the unruly forces of (female) nature (see Chapter 2 for a fuller discussion of this seventeenth-century cultural battle). Many critics invoked the image of Carson as an anti-science witch. The Vice Chancellor of the University of California/Riverside, Robert Metcalf, asked whether:

> [w]e are going to progress logically and scientifically upward, or whether we are going to drift back to the dark ages where witchcraft and witches reign . . . There are signs people do lean toward "witchery," and not only on the subject of pesticides. There are food faddists, and quacks in the medical field, and persons who oppose fluoridation of water.
> (cited in Hazlett, 2004, p. 707)

Other pesticide supporters also invoked the image of Carson as a witch. The cover of the October 1963 issue of the magazine *Farm Chemicals* featured a cartoon in which figures representing three industry spokesmen who testified before Congress forcefully make their case to Uncle Sam, one pounding the table with his fist, another pointing his finger in accusation, and the third gesturing thumbs down. Behind them, a witch on her broomstick flies by (image reproduced in Hazlett, 2004, p. 707).

Other criticism was equally ugly. Darby's *Chemical and Engineering News* review was titled "Silence, Miss Carson," tapping the cultural theme that women should know their place—which, the review was clearly suggesting, Carson didn't (Darby, 1962; see also Domosh and Seager, 2001). Other reviewers drew attention to Carson's "spinster" status (a close relative to a witch in popular cultural imaginary), suggesting that she was unworldly and bitter. Why was a "spinster . . . so worried about genetics?" former Agriculture Secretary Ezra Benson wondered.

Stigmatizing perfectly good chemicals* (*and killing Africans at the same time)

> *Died. DDT, age 95, a persistent pesticide and onetime humanitarian. Considered to be one of World War II's greatest heroes, DDT saw its reputation fade after it was charged with murder by author Rachel Carson. Death came on June 27 [1969] in Michigan after a lingering illness. Survived by dieldrin, aldrin, endrin, chlordane, heptachlor, lindane and toxaphene. Please omit flowers.*
> THE NEW YORK TIMES, 1969[6]

Following several state bans, including Michigan's in 1969, as described above, the EPA enacted a federal ban on DDT in 1972; or, rather, an incomplete ban because production for export was allowed to continue. Since then, worldwide, DDT's legal status and use has waxed and waned. The 2004 Stockholm Convention on POPs banned its use worldwide (for countries that signed the Convention), with exceptions made for its continued use in anti-malaria insect-control programs; by then, few countries were using it anyway. It continues to be widely used in India, and less so in China. The WHO on several occasions and for specific programs stopped using DDT for mosquito control because of insect resistance—wholesale spraying was becoming ineffective. But in 2007, the WHO and the parties to the Stockholm Convention cautiously restated their position that DDT could—and in some cases, should—still be used in a limited and controlled way, indoors, for insect control in the fight against disease, especially malaria (World Health Organization, 2011).

Carson never called for the banning of pesticides, warning instead about their overuse, misuse, and reckless use. She spent relatively little time in *Silent Spring* discussing DDT use in disease control (focusing primarily on its harm to wildlife and human health), but when she did, she lamented the astonishingly fast rise of insect resistance that ensured the futility of continued use of DDT:

> No responsible person contends that insect-borne disease should be ignored. The question that has now urgently presented itself is whether it is either wise or responsible to attack the problem by methods that are rapidly making it worse. The world has heard much of the triumphant war against disease through the control of insect vectors of infection, but it has heard little of the other side of the story—the defeats, the short-lived triumphs that now strongly support the alarming view that the insect enemy has been made actually stronger by our efforts. Even worse, we may have destroyed our very means of fighting.
>
> (pp. 234–235)

Carson was not directly involved in the US decision to ban DDT (which happened eight years after her death). She was not involved in decisions by the WHO to stop using DDT in some of their malaria programs because of insect resistance to it.

Nonetheless, the chemical industry's defenders (and producers) have never forgiven Carson—for many things, but especially for the end of the DDT era. In the late 1990s, conservatives in the United States launched a concerted effort to rehabilitate DDT and to indict Carson all over again.

In a remarkable twist, DDT has become a *cause célèbre* of the modern American conservative movement. Most analysts point to the work of a free-market, anti-regulatory economist, Roger Bate, as the catalyst for this movement. Bate is an ardent anti-environmentalist who shares the conservative ideological position that left-wing thinkers and activists distort science for their political ends—and that the conservatives are the protectors of "sound science." Bate (who is also a climate change denier) formulated a "Malaria Strategy" in the late 1990s, that he hoped would reveal the moral bankruptcy (in his view) of the modern environmental movement by revealing the ways in which environmental regulations harmed public health. The "perfect" case study that Bate seized on was the banning of DDT—which, he argued, could be seen as responsible for the resurgence of malaria in the poor world and thus the deaths of millions of people. Bate's critics suggest that he developed this strategy cynically, in an effort to deflect attention and funding away from the anti-tobacco movement that was then hitting full stride in the United States and Europe (Sarvana, 2009; Swartz, 2007). At the same time, this strategy allows conservatives to take another swipe at Rachel Carson, long their *bête noir.*

Bate helped to found the nonprofit Africa Fighting Malaria (AFM) to take the lead in his campaign. The AFM website contains a steady drumbeat of anti-Carson rhetoric, including stories such as "How Bad Science Opened the Door for Malaria," or "Demonizing DDT." One reprinted 2011 essay says baldly that:

In the US, a number of years ago, a woman, the late Rachel Carson, wrote a book called *Silent Spring*, which condemned DDT as being harmful to humans and to animals, particularly birds. This book was largely responsible for the large-scale banning of DDT all over the world. The book was wrong. In later life, Carson admitted that she had written it more as a novel than as a true scientific work, but the damage had been done. Millions of people had died as a result . . . There is now no evidence that would stand scientific scrutiny that shows that DDT is harmful to humans . . . When malaria was wiped out in Europe and the US in the mid 1970s, DDT was banned because of the claims of Carson et. al. They made African countries ban it too and the death rate in Africa soared. Meanwhile, the International Agency for Research on Cancer classifies DDT as a "possible carcinogen," which places it in the same category as beer, coffee and peanut butter. I am not aware of a single case in the world of any person getting cancer from DDT, and am certainly not aware of any deaths.

(Kemm, 2011)

The re-demonization of Carson has reached a fevered pitch. The Competitive Enterprise Institute (self-described as a free-market policy group that "addresses the dangers associated with anti-technology views, as embodied in Rachel Carson's *Silent Spring*") launched a website devoted entirely to anti-Carson activism: Rachel Was Wrong.[7] Conservatives have been remarkably successful at generating the notion that Carson had directly caused the DDT ban, and that the ban has directly caused the deaths of millions.

Anti-Carsonism has also reached the US government. In May 2007, Senator Tom Coburn (a Republican from Oklahoma) blocked a bill that would have named a post office in Springdale, Pennsylvania—Carson's birthplace—in her honor. The House had passed this bill, designated to mark Carson's 100th birthday, although in the House, 53 Republican Congressional representatives voted against it (including then-Minority, now Majority-Leader John Boehner). However, in the Senate, the bill was blocked entirely.[8] Coburn argued against memorializing Carson in her hometown, charging that Carson had "stigmatized" perfectly good chemicals, and that by working to ban harmful pesticides Carson was responsible for the deaths of millions of Africans. Coburn's statement reads:[9]

June 7, 2007

Dr. Coburn Stands for Science—Rachel Carson and the Death of Millions

Before the Congress left for Memorial Day recess, Dr. Coburn announced his intention to oppose unanimous passage of two bills intended to honor Rachel Carson on the 100th anniversary of her birth (one bill to name a post office after her in Pennsylvania, and a resolution honoring her). Carson was the author of the now-debunked Silent Spring, a book that was the catalyst in the deadly worldwide stigmatization against insecticides, especially DDT. DDT (sprayed in small, diluted amounts on the inside of houses) is the cheapest and most effective insecticide in the world for use in mosquito control. Mosquito bites lead to 500 million cases of malaria a year, 1–2 million of which are fatal. The majority of deaths are in tiny children and pregnant moms in Africa. The United States and western European countries all used DDT in the mid-20th century to eliminate malaria from their territories, but then banned the substance for use by poor countries today to combat their number one health threat.

Although the Stockholm Convention of 2000 (the international meeting that banned DDT) allowed for the use of DDT to fight public health threats, the stigma towards the chemical had by that time almost entirely eliminated its use. President Bush's new Malaria Initiative and the World Health Organization are now actively promoting DDT and other insecticides to save Africans from malaria.

Dr. Coburn opposes these measures honoring Carson because one tragic aspect of Carson's legacy is that unscientific DDT policies have led to, and continue to lead to, millions of preventable deaths in malaria-stricken countries.

Senator Coburn has kept this statement on his official website, now six years after the post office fight, and a link on the same website directs readers to the rachelwaswrong.org site. Carson had, by all accounts, a robust sense of humor; she might even be amused. But, most likely, she would be saddened by the obdurate insistence of her critics that the world can be saved by poisoning it.

Coda

The writer Margaret Atwood made Carson into a saint. In Atwood's dystopian novel, *The Year of the Flood*, "Saint Rachel of All Birds" is worshiped by a cult: God's Gardeners. The demonized Carson created by the right-wing in the United States, is as much a fiction as the be-sainted one created (tongue in cheek) by Atwood. But what is clearer than ever is that Carson—whoever we think she is—lives with us still.

As Margaret Atwood wrote in a 50th anniversary review of *Silent Spring*, many people turn to Carson's work still looking for answers:

> It's tempting to wonder what Carson would have done next had she lived. Would she have warned us that the human race was skirting the brink during the Vietnam war, when the fearsomely toxic herbicide, Agent Orange, was being shipped across the Pacific Ocean in huge vats to kill Vietnamese jungles? . . . what would Carson have said about the spraying of dispersants during the Gulf of Mexico oil spill? "Don't do it," no doubt. Many experts said this, but the powers that be did it anyway. What would she have said about the rapidly melting Arctic ice, or about the plans to shove a pipeline through the Great Bear rainforest to the Pacific shore [in Canada]?
>
> Our hi-tech civilization is leaking, and it's leaking into us. The more inventive we become, the longer grows the list of chemical compounds we may be breathing, eating and rubbing on to our skin. PCBs, chlorofluorocarbon refrigerants and dioxins have been identified and somewhat controlled, but many harmful chemicals

are still at large, and are joined every year by new ones we know little about.

Those [the 1950s–1960s] were less cynical times: people still trusted large corporations. Cigarette brands were still cosy household names ... Coca-Cola was still a synonym for wholesomeness ... Chemical companies were thought to be making life better every day, in every way, all over the world, which—to be fair—in some ways they were. Scientists in their white coats were presented as crusaders against the forces of ignorance and superstition, leading us forward under the banner of Discovery. Every modern scientific innovation was "progress" or "development", and progress and development were always desirable, and would march inevitably onward and upward: to question that belief was to question goodness, beauty and truth.

But now Carson was blowing the lid off. Had we been lied to, not only about pesticides, but about progress, and development, and discovery, and the whole ball of wax?

So one of the core lessons of *Silent Spring* was that things labelled progress weren't necessarily good. Another was that the perceived split between man and nature isn't real: the inside of your body is connected to the world around you, and your body too has its ecology, and what goes into it—whether eaten or breathed or drunk or absorbed through your skin—has a profound impact on you.

We're so used to thinking this way now that it's hard to imagine a time when general assumptions were different. But before Carson, they were.

(Atwood, 2012)

Notes

Introducing *Silent Spring*: Hitchcock, Bees, and the Syrian Civil War

1. http://www.valent.com/professional/products/safari/index.cfm (accessed July 23, 2013).
2. http://rt.com/usa/oregon-dead-bees-memorial-403/ (accessed July 23, 2013).
3. For the CBS coverage of this story, see http://www.cbsnews.com/news/organophosphate-pesticides-eyed-as-cause-of-india-poisonings-how-toxic/ (accessed February 12, 2014).
4. See Shiva (2006).
5. See *Silent Spring*, pp. 37–43.

1 Getting to *Silent Spring*

1. Nor was Cousteau's "silence" the same as Carson's—his was about the wonder and majesty of the "silent" deep sea; hers was about horror.
2. The Bureau was reorganized in 1940 to become the Fish and Wildlife Service.

2 The Post-War Machine in the Garden

1. The final title, *Silent Spring*, was suggested by Paul Brooks, but Carson was no doubt already predisposed to it. In the memorial page of the book, she cites Keats' poem, "La Belle Dame Sans Merci," the refrain of which is: "The sedge has withered from the lake,/And no birds sing."
2. The precarious position of women in science continues to be well documented. Two of the most prominent recent studies that

detail the particulars of this include: a 2012 study at Yale University, which revealed that science professors at American universities widely regard female undergraduates as less competent than male students with the same accomplishments and skills, and would pay them less if they were hiring (Moss-Racusin et al., 2012); a 1999 study at MIT of the status of women science faculty, which found widespread bias and marginalization (Committee on Women Faculty, 1999).

3   For a comprehensive study of the large dam era, see Billington et al. (2005).

4   Two reliable sources for information about US nuclear weapons testing are: Trinity Atomic Web Site at http://www.cddc.vt.edu/host/atomic/atmosphr/ustests.html, and Nuclear Weapons Archive at http://nuclearweaponarchive.org/Home.html

5   US Department of Justice: http://www.justice.gov/civil/common/reca.html

6   The Pugwash Conference takes its name from the location of the first meeting, which was held in 1957 in the village of Pugwash, Nova Scotia, Canada. For more information, see http://www.pugwash.org/

7   Carson much admired Muller and drew on his work for her own understanding of genetic mutations; Muller was one of Carson's most prominent defenders during the post-*Silent Spring* attacks on her.

8   The reports of the Federal Radiation Council are available on the website of the EPA: http://www.epa.gov/rpdweb00/federal/techdocs.html (accessed December 12, 2012).

9   A follow-up study in 2010, used a sample of the stored teeth from the original study: of those people in the sample who had died of cancer before the age of 50, all had strontium-90 (in their stored baby teeth) at significantly elevated levels compared with those who were still alive at age 50 (Mangano and Sherman, 2011). Other groups are using similar studies of baby teeth to detect contaminants, including the "Tooth Fairy" project in South Africa, tracing contaminants from mining operations.

10 For the official story of the Rocky Mountain Arsenal, see http://www.rma.army.mil/

11 See Carson, p. 18.

12 Compiled from several sources, including "Pesticide Products Registered for Use in New York State as of 1/2/2013": http://www.dec.ny.gov/chemical/27354.html

13 For some of the early scientific literature on Minamata disease in English-language science and medical journals, see: McAlpine and

Araki (1958); Takeuchi et al. (1959); McAlpine and Shukuro (1959) and Kurland et al. (1960).

14 The horrors of thalidomide fairly directly led to the eventual (partial) legalization of abortion in the United States. Sherry Finkbine, a well-known and loved figure on the TV show "Romper Room" took thalidomide—for morning sickness—that her husband brought back from England in 1962. When the bad news about thalidomide broke, Sherry's doctor recommended a "therapeutic abortion," the only kind of abortion then available in Arizona, where she lived. The hospital refused to provide the abortion and eventually Sherry flew to Sweden for it. The publicity over her struggle catalyzed public opinion in favor of legalizing abortion, and this is seen as a turning point in the establishment of a movement for abortion reform.

15 The author of the article on Kelsey interspersed his hard-hitting and otherwise serious review of her work with the same stereotypically sexist tropes used in most of the public media reviews of Carson, commenting on Kelsey's hair and dress style ("short hair, broad and flat heels"), her shyness, and her womanly skills (didn't like housework and wasn't a good cook).

3 Needless Havoc: Carson's Case Against Pesticides

1 A pesticide, according to the Environmental Protection Agency (EPA) in 2012, is defined as any substance or mixture of substances intended to prevent, destroy, repel, or mitigate any "pest." A "pest" is a living organism that occurs where it is not wanted or that causes damage to crops or humans or other animals. Examples include insects, rodents, other animals, unwanted plants ("weeds"), fungi, and microorganisms such as bacteria and viruses (see http://www.epa.gov/pesticides/about/index.htm). "Pesticides" is the umbrella category that includes insecticides, herbicides, fungicides, etc.

   In nature, of course, there is no such thing as a "pest"—this is a contrivance entirely of the human imagination.

2 The US Department of War, Film Bureau, film #195, "DDT – Weapon Against Disease" film and transcript are available at the US National Library of Medicines: http://collections.nlm.nih.gov/vplayer/vplayer.jsp?pid=nlm:nlmuid-9502511-vid (accessed February 2, 2013).

3 http://www.fws.gov/contaminants/Info/DDT.html

4 It should not be assumed that the US ban was an automatic outcome of the overwhelming scientific evidence of DDT's dangers.

The ban was hard-won and took place only after many court battles; it didn't ban the production of DDT for export from the United States, among other weaknesses.

5   The EPA technical factsheet on Chlordane is available at: http://www.epa.gov/pbt/pubs/chlordane.htm. The EPA "Basic Information about Heptachlor in Drinking Water" is available at: http://water.epa.gov/drink/contaminants/basicinformation/heptachlor.cfm. For the EPA Technology Transfer Network information on Air Toxics, see http://www.epa.gov/ttn/atw. For the Stockholm Convention list of the 12 initial POPs, see http://chm.pops.int/Convention/ThePOPs/The12InitialPOPs/tabid/296/Default.aspx. See also Natural Resources Defense Council: http://www.nrdc.org/breastmilk/hept.asp; EPA, http://blog.epa.gov/greeningtheapple/2013/06/30-years-after-the-epa-ban-chlordane-still-poisons-local-birds/

6   Ironically, but predictably, mosquitoes then developed resistance to dieldrin. A 1974 memo from the WHO field officers in Indonesia, detailed the back-and-forth applications between dieldrin and DDT that they were deploying to try to control malaria. Their report concludes with the sober assessment that mosquitoes will become resistant to whatever chemical is used, and that "naturalistic" methods of control were needed: http://apps.who.int/iris/bitstream/10665/65706/1/WHO_MAL_74.839.pdf

7   For the EPA Persistent Bioaccumulative and Toxic Chemical Program, information page on Aldrin/Dieldrin, see http://www.epa.gov/pbt/pubs/aldrin.htm. See also Toxic Substances and Disease Registry: http://www.atsdr.cdc.gov/toxfaqs/tf.asp?id=316&tid=56;

8   For more information, see Smithsonian National Zoological Park, Migratory Bird Center: http://nationalzoo.si.edu/scbi/migratorybirds/fact_sheets/default.cfm?fxsht=8 (accessed February 2, 2013).

9   Toxaphene is another one of the "dirty dozen" POPs outlawed by the Stockholm Convention. It was used primarily in the south, from 1947 to 1980, on cotton fields, and was one of the most heavily used insecticides in the United States.

10 http://www.epa.gov/opp00001/factsheets/legisfac.htm; correspondence with the EPA Pesticides Customer Service, February 27, 2013.

11 http://www.epa.gov/oppt/existingchemicals/pubs/tscainventory/basic.html#what

12 A "pesticide product" is the final brand that is sold on the market. Each pesticide product consists of "active ingredients," which are the chemicals that do the active work of the pesticide, killing or controlling the pest, and "inert" ingredients that may be more or less

harmful in themselves but that do not do the active work of the pesticide.

13 New York: http://www.dec.ny.gov/chemical/27354.html; Florida: http://www.flpesticide.us; Illinois: http://www.agr.state.il.us/Environment/Pesticide/productsearch.php; Michigan: http://state.ceris.purdue.edu/htbin/stweb.com

14 In bird killings related to new chemical introductions, but not pesticidal, vulture populations in the Indian subcontinent dropped by 95 percent between 2000 and 2003 due to the new introduction of diclofenac, an anti-inflammatory veterinarian drug that became a popular treatment for livestock—vultures died after scavenging carcasses of livestock containing diclofenac residues.

15 CNN: http://edition.cnn.com/search/?query=pesticide&x=0&y=0&primaryType=mixed&sortBy=relevance&intl=false#&sortBy=date; *New York Times*: http://query.nytimes.com/search/sitesearch/#/archives

4 One in Every Four

1 See, for example, Jenkins (1994) and Steinberg (2006).

2 See DeBug the Myths: http://debugthemyths.com/index.php?option=com_content&view=article&id=2&Itemid=3 (accessed February 2, 2013).

3 Lindane is a neurotoxin pesticide, banned for agricultural use in the 2009 round of Stockholm Convention agreements; however, the lindane agreement includes a pharmaceutical exemption, allowing for its continuing use in personal products (shampoo, creams) for lice and scabies control. Lindane products continue to be available in the United States by prescription, although its use has dropped considerably.

4 Interested readers might look at some news analysis such as "Testosterone and high finance do not mix," *The Observer* (UK), June 18, 2011; or several of the chapters in Enloe (2013).

5 For an excellent biography of Stewart, see Greene (1999).

6 Explanations of the regulatory system can be found at the EPA site http://www.epa.gov/pesticides/factsheets/securty.htm (accessed February 1, 2013) and the USDA at http://www.ams.usda.gov/AMSv1.0/pdp (accessed February 1, 2013). The USDA also provides an annual report of the pesticide residues found in the food supply. A contemporary critique of the food residue testing system is available through the "Pesticide Action Network": http://www.

panna.org/issues/food-agriculture/pesticides-on-food (accessed February 12, 2013).
7 http://www.gao.gov/products/GAO-11-289
8 http://www.ewg.org/foodnews/summary.php
9 http://www.fda.gov/downloads/Food/FoodborneIllnessContaminants/Pesticides/UCM352872.pdf
10 For more information, see World Wildlife Fund (1998).
11 Centers for Disease Control: http://www.cdc.gov/injury/wisqars/leadingcauses.html
12 For more information, see the Natural Resources Defense Council: http://www.nrdc.org/health/effects/bendrep.asp (accessed February 2, 2013).

5 Alternatives

1 http://www.epa.gov/pesticides/factsheets/ipm.htm – content
2 "Citizen science" may have "arrived," but it is still resisted and denigrated by many in the formal sciences, and the usefulness of amateurs and amateur observations to science is highly contested. The contestation is often gendered, as female community activists confront male experts. For a discussion of this dynamic, see, for example, Seager (1996).
3 For background papers and the full text of the precautionary principle, see http://www.sehn.org/precaution.html. See also http://www.silentspring.org/faqs/precautionary-principle (both accessed February 2, 2013).

6 Responses to *Silent Spring*

1 International details from http//www.environmentandsociety.org/exhibitions/silent-spring/silent-spring-international-best-seller
2 The full PSAC report is available at http://timpanogos.wordpress.com/2012/12/10/use-of-pesticides-report-of-the-presidents-science-advisory-committee-may–15–1963/ (accessed July 10, 2013).
3 See, http://www.environmentandsociety.org/exhibitions/silent-spring/us-federal-government-responds
4 The Monsanto brochure is available for download from the website of the International Society for Environmental Ethics: http://

enviroethics.org/2011/12/02/the-desolate-year-monsanto-magazine–1962/ (accessed February 2, 2013).

5   The tactic of casting women environmentalists as "hysterical" continues today (see Seager, 1996).
6   An "obituary" written by Hall Higdon for DDT in the aftermath of Michigan banning all sales (due to mounting evidence of extremely high concentrations in the food chain and a threat to the salmon fishery). See Higdon (1969).
7   http://rachelwaswrong.org
8   The bill eventually passed in 2008.
9   See http://www.coburn.senate.gov/public/index.cfm/rightnow?ContentRecord_id=16ea56f1–5c06–4e30–965e-ca7e91034178&ContentType_id=b4672ca4–3752–49c3-bffc-fd099b51c966&Group_id=00380921–999d–40f6-a8e3–470468762340

Sources for Further Reading and Research

On Rachel Carson

Brooks, P. (1972), *The House of Life: Rachel Carson at Work*. New York: Houghton Mifflin.
Environment and Society Portal: http://www.environmentandsociety.org/search?search_api_views_fulltext=rachel+carson
Freeman, M. (ed.) (1995), *Always, Rachel: The Letters of Rachel Carson and Dorothy Freeman, 1952–1964*. Boston: Beacon Press.
Lear, L. (2009),. *Rachel Carson: Witness for Nature*. Boston, NY: Houghton Mifflin.
Rachel Carson.org: http://www.rachelcarson.org/AboutLinda.aspx
Rachel Carson Institute, Chatham College: http://www.chatham.edu/rachelcarson/
Rachel Carson National Wildlife Refuge: http://www.fws.gov/refuge/rachel_carson/

On *Silent Spring* and responses to it

Graham, Jr., F. (1970), *Since Silent Spring*. Boston: Houghton Mifflin.
Hazlett, M. (2004), "Woman vs. man vs. bugs: Gender and popular ecology in early reactions to *Silent Spring*," *Environmental History* 9(4): 701–729.
Hynes, P. (1989), *The Recurring Silent Spring*. New York: Pergamon Press.
Lear, L. (1992), "Bombshell in Beltsville: The USDA and the challenge of Silent Spring," *Agricultural History* 66(2): 151–170.

Smith, M. B. (2001), "'Silence, Miss Carson!' Science, Gender, and the Reception of *Silent Spring*," *Feminist Studies*, 27(3): 733–752.

On pesticides today

Environmental Protection Agency: http://www.epa.gov/pesticides/
Pesticide Action Network: http://www.panna.org/
USDA. "Pesticide Data Program—Annual Summaries:" http://www.ams.usda.gov/AMSv1.0/ams.fetchTemplateData.do?template=TemplateG&topNav=&leftNav=ScienceandLaboratories&page=PDPDownloadData/Reports&description=Download+PDP+Data/Reports&acct=pestcddataprg

On environmental and health threats

Agency for Toxic Substances and Disease Registry: http://www.atsdr.cdc.gov/substances/index.asp
Centers for Disease Control and Prevention (US), Environmental Health Program: http://www.cdc.gov/environmental/
Colborn, T., Dumanoski, D., and Myers, J. P. (1996), *Our Stolen Future*. New York: Plume/Penguin.
National Institute of Environmental Health Sciences (US): http://www.niehs.nih.gov/
Oreskes, N. and Conway, E. (2010), *Merchants of Doubt*. New York, London: Bloomsbury Press.
President's Cancer Panel Annual Report, 2008–2009, "Reducing Environmental Cancer Risk". Released April 2010. Bethesda MD: National Institutes of Health.
Seager, J. (1993), *Earth Follies: Coming to Feminist Terms with the Global Environmental Crisis*. New York: Routledge; London: Earthscan.
Shulman, S. (1992), *The Threat at Home: Confronting the Toxic Legacy of the US Military*. Boston: Beacon Press.
Silent Spring Institute: http://www.silentspring.org/
Steingraber, S. (1997), *Living Downstream*. New York: Random House.

Bibliography

Adams, C. J. (1990), *The Sexual Politics of Meat: A Feminist-Vegetarian Critical Theory*. New York: Continuum.
Atwood, M. (2012), "Rachel Carson's *Silent Spring*, 50 years on." *The Guardian*, December 7. http://www.guardian.co.uk/books/2012/dec/07/why-rachel-carson-is-a-saint (accessed February 4, 2013).
Balsamo, A. (1996), *Technologies of the Gendered Body: Reading Cyborg Women*. Durham and London: Duke University Press.
Billington, D., Jackson, D., and Martin, M. (2005), *The History of Large Federal Dams: Planning, Design, and Construction in the Era of Big Dams*. Denver, CO: US Department of Interior, Bureau of Reclamation.
Brinkley, D. (2012), "Rachel Carson and JFK, An environmental tag team." *Audubon Magazine*, May–June. http://www.audubonmagazine.org/articles/conservation/rachel-carson-and-jfk-environmental-tag-team (accessed July 10, 2013).
Brooks, P. (1972), *The House of Life: Rachel Carson at Work*. New York: Houghton Mifflin.
Calvert, G., Karnik, J., Mehler, L., Beckman, J., Morrissey, B., Sievert, J., Barrett, R., and Moraga-McHaley, S. (2008), "Acute pesticide poisoning among agricultural workers in the United States, 1998–2005." *American Journal of Industrial Medicine* 51: 883–898.
Carson, R. (1941), *Under the Sea-wind*. New York: Oxford University Press
Carson, R. (1951), *The Sea Around Us*. New York: Oxford University Press
Carson, R. (1955), *The Edge of the Sea*. Boston: Houghton Mifflin Company.
Carson, R. (1963), "Environmental hazards: Control of pesticides and other chemical poisons." Statement of Rachel Carson before the Subcommittee on Reorganization and International Organizations of the Committee on Government Operations, June 4. http://www.rachelcarsoncouncil.org/index.php?page=rachel-carson-s-statement-before-congress--1963 (accessed August 4, 2013).
Carson, R. (1967), *Silent Spring* (5th Fawcett Press printing). New York: Fawcett Crest. (Original work published 1962.)

Carson, R. (1998a), *The Sense of Wonder*. New York: Harper Collins. (Original work published 1965.)
Carson, R. (1998b), *Lost Woods: The Discovered Writing of Rachel Carson*. Ed. L. Lear. Boston: Beacon Press.
Centers for Disease Control and Prevention (CDC). (2009), *Fourth National Report on Human Exposures to Environmental Chemicals*. Atlanta, GA: US Department of Health and Human Services Centers for Disease Control and Prevention.
Cockburn, C. (1983), *Brothers: Male Dominance and Technological Change*. London: Pluto.
Cockburn, C. and Ormrod, S. (1993), *Gender and Technology in the Making*. London: Sage.
Colborn, T., Dumanoski, D., and Myers, J. P. (1996), *Our Stolen Future*. New York: Plume/Penguin.
Committee on Women Faculty in the School of Science. (1999), "A study on the status of women faculty in science at MIT." Cambridge, MA: MIT. http://web.mit.edu/fnl/women/women.html (accessed December 20, 2012).
Daemmrich, A. (2002), "A tale of two experts: Thalidomide and political engagement in the United States and West Germany." *Social History of Medicine* 151(1): 137–158.
Darby, W. J. (1962), "Silence, Miss Carson." *Chemical and Engineering News* 40 (October 1): 60–63.
Del Tredici, R. (1987), *At Work in the Fields of the Bomb*. New York: Harper & Row.
Delaplane, K. (1996), *Pesticide Usage in the United States: History, Benefits, Risks and Trends*. Athens, GA: Cooperative Extension Service, The University of Georgia.
Domosh, M. and Seager, J. (2001), *Putting Women in Place: Feminist Geographers Make Sense of the World*. New York: Guilford Press.
Donovan, J. (1990), "Animal rights and feminist theory." *Signs* 15(2) (Winter): 350–375.
Dreier, P. (2012), *The 100 Greatest Americans of the 20th Century*. New York: Nation Books.
Drew, E. (1970), "Dam outrage." *Atlantic Monthly* 225 (April): 51–62.
Dunlap, T. (1981), *DDT: Scientists, Citizens, and Public Policy*. Princeton, NJ: Princeton University Press.
Easlea, B. (1983), *Fathering the Unthinkable: Masculinity, Scientists and the Nuclear Arms Race*. London: Pluto Press.
Eddleston, M., Buckley, N. A., Eyer, P., and Dawson, A. H. (2008), "Management of acute organophosphorus pesticide poisoning." *Lancet* 371(9612): 597–607.
Eiseley, L. (1962), "Using a plague to fight a plague." *The Saturday Review*, September 29.

BIBLIOGRAPHY

Eisenhower, Dwight D. (1961), Farewell address to the nation. January 17. Information Clearing House. Transcript available at http://www.informationclearinghouse.info/article5407.htm (accessed December 12, 2012).

Elliott, D. B., Krivickas, K., Brault, M. W., and Kreider, R. M. (2012), "Historical marriage trends from 1890–2010: A focus on race differences." Annual meeting of the Population Association of America. SEHSD Working Paper Number 2012–12. http://paa2012.princeton.edu/abstracts/121083 (accessed December 12, 2012).

Emel, J. (1995), "Are you man enough, big and bad enough? Ecofeminism and wolf eradication in the USA." *Environment and Planning D: Society and Space* 13(6): 707–734.

Enloe, C. (2000), *Maneuvers: The International Politics of Militarizing Women's Lives.* Berkeley, CA: University of California Press.

Enloe, C. (2002), "Sneak attack: The militarization of U.S. culture." *Ms* 15 (December/January).

Enloe, C. (2013), *Seriously! Investigating Crashes and Crises as if Women Matter.* Berkeley, CA: University of California Press.

EnviroNews Forum. (1999), "Killer environment." *Environmental Health Perspectives* 107(2): A62.

Faderman, L. (1981), *Surpassing the Love of Men.* New York: Morrow and Company.

Faludi, S. (1991), *Backlash: The Undeclared War Against American Women.* New York: Anchor Books, Doubleday.

Fleming, J. R. (2010), *Fixing the Sky: The Checkered History of Weather and Climate Control.* New York: Columbia University Press.

Foster, J. B. and Clark, B. (2008), "Rachel Carson's ecological critique." *Monthly Review* 59(9): 1–17.

Freeman, M. (ed.) (1995), *Always, Rachel: The Letters of Rachel Carson and Dorothy Freeman.* Boston: Beacon Press.

Gilliam, C. (2012), "Genetically modified crops have led to pesticide increase, study finds." *Huffington Post*, October 10. http://www.huffingtonpost.com/2012/10/02/genetically-modified-crops-pesticides_n_1931020.html (accessed February 2, 2013).

Government Accountability Office (GAO). (1990), *Lawn Care Pesticide Risks and Prohibited Safety Claims.* GAO/RCED-90–134. Washington, DC: Government Printing Office.

Government Accountability Office (GAO). (2009), *High-risk Series: An Update.* GAO-09–271. Washington, DC: Government Printing Office.

Greene, G. (1999), *The Woman Who Knew Too Much.* Ann Arbor: University of Michigan Press.

Grey, S. (2008), "In defense of Rachel Carson." *International Socialist Review* 57 (Jan–Feb). http://www.isreview.org/issues/57/57.shtml (accessed February 20, 2013).

Griswold, E. (2012), "The wild life of 'Silent Spring'." *New York Times*, September 23. http://query.nytimes.com/gst/fullpage.html?res=9802EFD81030F930A1575AC0A9649D8B63 (accessed December 12, 2012).

Grunwald, M. (2006), *The Swamp: The Everglades, Florida, and the Politics of Paradise*. New York: Simon & Schuster.

Gunnell, D. and Eddleston, M. (2003), "Suicide by intentional ingestion of pesticides: A continuing tragedy in developing countries." *International Journal of Epidemiology* 32(6): 902–909.

Hacker, S. (1989), *Pleasure, Power and Technology: Some Tales of Gender, Engineering, and the Cooperative Workplace*. New York: Routledge.

Harada, M., Hanada, M., Tajiri, M., Inoue, Y., Hotta, N., Fujino, T., Takaoka, S., and Ueda, K. (2011), "Mercury pollution in First Nations Groups in Ontario, Canada: 35 years of Canadian Minamata Disease." *Journal of Minamata Studies* 3: 3–30.

Harding, S. (1986), *The Science Question in Feminism*. Ithaca, NY: Cornell University Press.

Harding, S. (1997), "Women's standpoints on nature: What makes them possible?" *Osiris* 12 (2nd Series), Women, Gender, and Science: New Directions: 186–200.

Hazlett, M. (2004, October), "Woman vs. man vs. bugs: Gender and popular ecology in early reactions to *Silent Spring*." *Environmental History* 9(4): 701–729.

Hazlett, M. (2008), "Science and spirit: Struggles of the early Rachel Carson." In L. Sideris and K. D. Moore (eds), *Rachel Carson: Legacy and Challenge*. New York: State University of New York Press.

Higdon, H. (1969), "Obituary for DDT (in Michigan)." *New York Times*, July 6.

Horkheimer, M. (1985), *Eclipse of Reason*. New York: Continuum. (Original work published 1947.)

Human Events. (2005), "Ten most harmful books of the 19th and 20th centuries." Human Events: Powerful Conservative Voices. http://www.humanevents.com/2005/05/31/ten-most-harmful-books-of-the–19th-and–20th-centuries/ (accessed December 12, 2012).

Hynes, P. (1989), *The Recurring Silent Spring*. New York: Pergamon Press.

Jackson-Houlston, C. (2006), "'Queen lilies'? The interpenetration of scientific, religious and gender discourses in Victorian representations of plants." *Journal of Victorian Culture* 11(1): 84–110. http://muse.jhu.edu/journals/journal_of_victorian_culture/v011/11.1jackson_houlston.html (accessed December 12, 2012).

Janzen, M. (2010), "The cranberry scare of 1959." PhD dissertation, Texas A&M University.

Jenkins, V. S. (1994), *The Lawn: A History of an American Obsession*. Washington, DC: Smithsonian Institution Press.

Jenks, A. (2010), "The Minamata disease and the true costs of Japanese modernization." In *Perils of Progress: Environmental Disasters in the 20th Century*. New York: Pearson.

Johnson, S. (1947), "Farm science and citizens." In United States Department of Agriculture, *The Yearbook of Agriculture 1943–1947: Science in Farming*. Washington, DC: US Government Printing Office.

Jones, J. (2011), "Americans most confident in military, least in Congress." Gallup Poll, June 23. http://www.gallup.com/poll/148163/americans-confident-military-least-congress.aspx

Keller, E. (1985), *Reflections on Gender and Science*. New Haven: Yale University Press.

Kemm, K. (2011), "DDT, a potent weapon against malaria." *AFM News*, 20 May. http://www.fightingmalaria.org/news.aspx?id=1627 (accessed February 20, 2013).

Kreiger, R. (2005), "Reviewing some origins of pesticide perceptions." *Outlooks on Pest Management* 16: 244–248.

Kurland, T., Faro, S. N., and Siedler, H. (1960), "Minamata disease: The outbreak of a neurologic disorder in Minamata, Japan, and its relationship to the ingestion of seafood contaminated by mercuric compounds." *World Neurology* 1(5): 370–395.

Lear, L. (1992), "Bombshell in Beltsville: The USDA and the challenge of Silent Spring." *Agricultural History* 66(2) (Spring): 151–170.

Lear, L. (1993), "Rachel Carson's *Silent Spring*." *Environmental History Review* 17(2): 23–48. http://www.history.vt.edu/Barrow/Hist3706/readings/lear.html (accessed November 22, 2013).

Lear, L. (2009), *Rachel Carson: Witness for Nature*. Boston and New York: Houghton Mifflin.

Leiss, W. (1972), *The Domination of Nature*. Montreal: McGill-Queen's University.

Leiss, W. (2007), "Modern science, enlightenment, and the domination of nature: no exit?" *Fast Capitalism*. http://www.uta.edu/huma/agger/fastcapitalism/2_2/leiss.html (accessed December 12, 2012).

Leonard, J. (1951), ". . . And his wonders in the deep." *New York Times*, July 1.

Lovelock, J. E. (1979), *Gaia: A New Look at Life on Earth*. Oxford: Oxford University Press.

Mangano, J. and Sherman, J. (2011), "Elevated *in vivo* strontium-90 from nuclear weapons fallout among cancer decedents: A case-control study of deciduous teeth." *International Journal of Health Services* 41(1): 137–158.

Marx, K. (1973), *Grundrisse: Foundations of the Critique of Political Economy*. New York: Vintage Books. (Original work published 1939.)

Marx, L. (1956), "The Machine in the Garden." *The New England Quarterly* 29(1): 27–42.

Marx, L. (1999), *The Machine in the Garden: Technology and the Pastoral Ideal in America*. New York: Oxford University Press. (Original work published 1964.)

McAlpine, D. and Araki, S. (1958), "Minamata disease: An unusual neurological disorder caused by contaminated fish." *Lancet* 2(7047): 629.

McAlpine, D. and Shukuro, A. (1959), "Minamata disease: Late effects of an unusual neurological disorder caused by contaminated fish." *Archives of Neurology* 1(5): 522.

McKibben, B. (1990), *The End of Nature*. London: Penguin.

Merchant, C. (1980), *The Death of Nature: Women, Ecology, and the Scientific Revolution*. San Francisco: Harper Collins.

Merchant, C. (1983), "Out of the past: Women, nature, and domination." In J. Zimmerman (ed.), *Future, Technology, and Woman*. New York: Praeger.

Merchant, C. (2003), *Reinventing Eden: The Fate of Nature in Western Culture*. New York: Routledge.

Merchant, C. (2006), "The scientific revolution and the *Death of Nature*." *Isis* 97: 513–533.

Merchant, C. (2008), "'The violence of impedinents': Francis Bacon and the origins of experimentation." *Isis* 99: 731–760

Merchant, C. (2010), "Environmentalism: From the control of nature to partnership." University of California Bernard Moses Lecture, May 4. Transcript available at http://nature.berkeley.edu/merchant (accessed December 12, 2012).

Messier, S. (2012), "Research findings: Rachel L. Carson and 'the sea around us'." http://www.squidinkbooks.com/rachel-carson.htm (accessed December 21, 2012).

Michaels, D. (2008), *Doubt is Their Product*. Oxford: Oxford University Press.

Mies, M. and Shiva, V. (1993), *Ecofeminism*. London: Zed Books.

Moss-Racusin, C. A., Dovidio, J.F., Brescoll, V. L., Grahama, M. J., and Handelsman, J. (2012), "Science faculty's subtle gender biases favor male students." *Proceedings of the National Academy of Sciences* 109(41): 16474–16479.

Mulliken, J. (1962), "The woman doctor who would not be hurried." *Life Magazine* 53 (10 August): 28–29.

Mustard, D. (2000), "Spinster: An evolving stereotype revealed through film." *Journal of Media Psychology*, January 20. http://www.calstatela.edu/faculty/sfischo/spinster.html (accessed December 20, 2012).

National Institute for Minamata Disease. (2012), Minamata disease archives. http://www.nimd.go.jp/archives/english/index.html (accessed December 12, 2012).

National Pesticide Information Center. (1999), "DDT: General fact sheet." Oregon State University.
Noble, D. (1991), *A World Without Women: The Evolution of the Masculine Culture of Science*. New York: Knopf.
O'Brien, W. (2007), "Continuity in a changing environmental discourse: Film depictions of Corps of Engineers projects in South Florida." *Geojournal* 69: 135–149.
Oelschlaeger, M. (1993), *The Idea of Wilderness from Prehistory to the Age of Ecology*. New Haven: Yale University Press.
Oldenziel, R. (1999), *Making Technology Masculine: Men, Women and Modern Machines in America*. Amsterdam: Amsterdam University Press.
Oreskes, N. and Conway, E. (2010), *Merchants of Doubt*. New York, London: Bloomsbury.
Pattberg, P. (2007), "Conquest, domination, and control: Europe's mastery of nature in historic perspective." *Journal of Political Ecology* 14(1): 9.
Pesticide Action Network. (2004), *Chemical Trespass: Pesticides in Our Bodies and Corporate Accountability*. San Francisco: PAN.
Plass, G. N. (1956), "Carbon dioxide and the climate." *American Scientist* 44: 302–316.
Plumwood, V. (1993), *Feminism and the Mastery of Nature*. New York: Routledge.
Reiss, L. Z. (1961), "Strontium-90 absorption by deciduous teeth." *Science* 134: 1669–1673.
Rossiter, M. (1998), *Women Scientists in America: Before Affirmative Action, 1940–1972*. Baltimore: Johns Hopkins University Press.
Sarvana, A. (2009), "Bate and switch: How a free-market magician manipulated two decades of environmental science." *Natural Resources News Service*, June 2. http://www.storiesthatmatter.org/20090602105/natural-resources-news-service/bate-and-switch-how-a-free-market-magician-manipulated-two-decades-of-environmental-science.html (accessed February 28, 2013).
Saturday Review (1962a), "The unfinished story of thalidomide," September 1, p. 35
Saturday Review (1962b), "Where is science taking us?" September 1, pp. 44–5.
Schneider, K. (1991), "Military has new strategic goal in cleanup of vast toxic waste." *New York Times*, August 15, p. A1.
Seager, J. (1993a), *Earth Follies: Coming to Feminist Terms with the Global Environmental Crisis*. New York: Routledge.
Seager, J. (1993b), "A not-so-natural disaster: How military-think gave rise to the great Mississippi flood of 1993." *MS. Magazine*, Nov/Dec, 26–27.

Seager, J. (1996), "Hysterical housewives and other mad women: Grassroots environmental organizing in the USA." In D. Rocheleau, E. Wangari, and B. Thomas-Slater (eds), *Toward a Feminist Political Ecology: Global Perspectives from Local Experience*. New York: Routledge.

Seager, J. (1999), "Patriarchal vandalism: Militaries and the environment." In J. Silliman and Y. King (eds), *Dangerous Intersections: Feminist Perspectives on Population, Environment and Development*. Cambridge: South End Press, pp. 163–188.

Seager, J. (2003), "Rachel Carson died of breast cancer: Feminist environmentalism comes of age." *SIGNS* 28(3): 945–972.

Shiva, S. (2006), "India drowning in pesticides." *CBS News*, 16 August. http://www.cbsnews.com/news/organophosphate-pesticides-eyed-as-cause-of-india-poisonings-how-toxic/ (accessed July 18, 2013).

Shiva, V. (1988), *Staying Alive: Women, Ecology and Development*. London: Zed Books.

Shteir, A. (1997), "Gender and modern botany in Victorian England." *Osiris* (2nd Series) 12, Women, Gender, and Science: New Directions: 29–38.

Shulman, S. (1992), *The Threat at Home: Confronting the Toxic Legacy of the US Military*. Boston: Beacon Press.

Smith, M. B. (2001), "Silence, Miss Carson! Science, gender, and the reception of *Silent Spring*." *Feminist Studies* 27(3) (Autumn): 733–752.

State of New Jersey. (2008), "Hazardous substance fact sheet, 2,4-D." http://nj.gov/health/eoh/rtkweb/documents/fs/0593.pdf (accessed February 2, 2013).

Steingraber, S. (2008), "Living downstream of *Silent Spring*." In L. Sideris and K. D. Moore (eds), *Rachel Carson: Legacy and Challenge*. New York: State University of New York Press.

Steinberg, T. (2006), *American Green: The Obsessive Quest for the Perfect Lawn*. New York: W.W. Norton & Co.

Stoll, M. (2012), "Industrial and agricultural interests fight back." Environment and Society Portal. http://www.environmentandsociety.org/exhibitions/silent-spring/industrial-and-agricultural-interests-fight-back (accessed February 12, 2013).

Swartz, A. (2007), "Rachel Carson, mass murderer?" Fairness and Accuracy in Reporting (FAIR), September 1. http://fair.org/extra-online-articles/Rachel-Carson,-Mass-Murderer/ (accessed February 27, 2013).

Swerdlow, A. (1993), *Women Strike for Peace*. Chicago: The University of Chicago Press.

Takeuchi, T., Kambara, T., Morikawa, N., Matsumoto, H., Shiraishi, Y., and Ito, H. (1959), "Pathologic observations of the Minamata Disease." *Pathology International* 9: 769–783.

BIBLIOGRAPHY

Taylor, P. (1986), *Respect for Nature: A Theory of Environmental Ethics*. Princeton: Princeton University Press.
The Japan Times. (2012),. "Lucky dragon's lethal catch," March 18. http://www.japantimes.co.jp/text/fl20120318x1.html (accessed February 20, 2013).
The New York Times (1962), "Doctor's action bars birth defects", July 16, p. 24.
The New York Times. (1964),. "Obituary: Rachel Carson dies of cancer," April 15. http://www.nytimes.com/books/97/10/05/reviews/carsonobit.html (accessed December 12, 2012).
Time. (1953),. "Science: Invisible blanket," May 25. http://www.time.com/time/magazine/article/00,9171,890597,00.html?promoid=googlep (accessed December 12, 2012).
Toossi, M. (2002), "A century of change: The US labor force, 1950–2050." *Monthly Labor Review* 125: 15–28.
Trost, C. (1984), *Elements of Risk: The Chemical Industry and its Threat To America*. New York: Times Books.
USDA. (2011), *Pesticide Data Program—Annual Summary, Calendar Year 2011*. Washington, DC: USDA.
USEPA. (1975), "DDT regulatory history: A brief survey (to 1975)." http://www.epa.gov/aboutepa/history/topics/ddt/02.html (accessed February 1, 2013).
USEPA. (2011), *Pesticides Industry Sales and Usage: 2006 and 2007 Market Estimates*. Washington, DC: Office of Pesticide Programs.
US News & World Report (1962), "New Drugs—How Good are the Safeguards?" August 13, pp. 56–7.
Van den Berg, H. (2008), "Global status of DDT and its alternatives for use in vector control to prevent disease." Background report for UNEP "Stakeholders' Meeting to review the interim report for the establishment of a global partnership to develop alternatives to DDT. Geneva, November 3–5.
Wajcman, J. (1991), *Feminism Confronts Technology*. London: Polity Press.
Walker, K. and Walsh, L. (2012), "'No one yet knows what the ultimate consequences may be': How Rachel Carson transformed scientific uncertainty into a site for public participation." *Journal of Business and Technical Communication* 26(1): 3–34.
Warren, K. (2000), *Ecofeminist Philosophy: A Western Perspective on What it is and why it Matters*. New York: Rowman & Littlefield.
Will, J. "The Feminine Conscience of FDA." *Saturday Review*, September 1, 42.
World Health Organization (WHO). (2011), *The Use of DDT in Malaria Vector Control*. Geneva: World Health Organization.
World Wildlife Fund. (1998), "Resolving the DDT dilemma: Protecting biodiversity and human health." http://wwf.panda.org/?4105/

resolvingthe-ddt-dilemma-protecting-biodiversity-and-human-health-wwfjune–1998 (accessed March 24, 2014).

Yip, P. and Liu, K. (2006), "The ecological fallacy and the gender ratio of suicide in China." *The British Journal of Psychiatry* 189: 465–466.

Zimmer, C. (2010), "Answers begin to emerge on how Thalidomide caused defects." *New York Times*, March 15, D3.

Index

accumulating sequence of poisoning 51, 52, 74, 75–77, 131
"act now, worry later" mentality 154
activism
　anti-Carson 169
　breast cancer activism 136
　Carson collected reports from activist groups 68
　citizen science 151
　the Long Island spraying case 150–151
acute vs chronic pesticide poisoning (human) 99, 119, 120, 133 *see also* low-level effects of pesticides
aerial spraying programs
　acute vs chronic effects 120
　aldrin in Detroit 94
　Carson particularly against 69–71, 89–92
　and citizen science ("letters-from-readers") 151
　and the exaggerated need for control 38–39
　fire ant eradication programs 38–39, 69–70, 79, 91
　Florida salt marsh spraying 97
　garden spraying devices 114
　gypsy moth spraying programs 38–39, 56, 70, 91–92, 150–151
　herbicides and the sagelands 87
　as last resort in IPM (integrated pest management) 149
　Miramichi region 96–98
　multiple spray runs on the same area 92
　and "pesticide drift" 89, 90–92, 103
　proved efficacious in WWII 73
　selective spraying 149–150
　in Sheldon, Illinois 88–89
　triggers for the book 69–70
　and ubiquitousness of poisons in food 121
　and WWII surplus planes 55
Africa Fighting Malaria 168
Africans, Carson held responsible for deaths of 168–170
agricultural practices, changing instead of pesticide use 93 *see also* biological control
Agricultural Research Service (ARS) 162
agricultural workers, threat to 79, 81, 99, 103, 105, 132–133
airborne contamination *see also* aerial spraying programs
　air currents transport thousands of miles 82
　"Lucky Dragon" catastrophe 47–48
　strontium-90 50
　unpredictability of wind transfer 51
　"white granular powder" 24, 50
aldrin 72, 77, 82, 88–89, 94, 162

amateur scientists 150–152
American Dream 112–113
American Medical Association (AMA) 37, 69, 113
aminotriazole and the cranberry crisis 59–60
anger, Carson showing 85
animals, testing on 122
anti-environmentalism 168
anti-science, Carson not 144, 165
anti-tobacco movement 168
anti-vivisection 90
apples 105
aquatic environments
 bioaccumulation in food chain 76
 Carson on 96–98
 half-lives of chemicals are longer than in soil 77
Army Corps of Engineers 41–42
arrogance
 Carson sees attempts to control nature as 25–26
 nuclear power and pesticide power derive from "man's" 53
Arsenal, Rocky Mountain 53–54
atomic world 41–58
attacks (on *Silent Spring*)
 Carson expected attacks from industry leaders 83
 Carson lived long enough to experience 2
 on Carson's science 163
 from chemical industry 159–163
 continuing today 7, 166–170
 counter-evidence of benefits of pesticides 163–164
 indirectly assisted by USDA 163
 personal attacks on Carson as a woman 164
attacks on Stewart's work on X-rays 119
Atwood, Margaret 171–172
Auerbach, Charlotte 139

authoritarianism 34, 118
avitrol 104
awareness
 awareness raising 140
 Carson's goal of education 34–35, 36, 83, 138, 150–152
 citizen science 36, 150–152
 inattention (of citizens) 34–35, 118
 public awareness and *Silent Spring* 160–163
 unawareness of most people 144
 willful ignorance 154

babies
 birth deformities in Minamata 61, 62
 pesticide residues in baby food 125
 pesticides in breastmilk 68, 118
 potential damage from X-rays 119
 and thalidomide 63–66
 transmission from mother to child 74, 118
baby teeth study 50
Bacon, Francis/Baconian science 27–28, 29, 32, 57, 67, 165
balance of nature 85, 147, 165
banned chemicals 5, 78, 80, 82, 162, 166–167, 168
BASF 99, 103
Bate, Roger 167–168
Bayer 4, 99
beauty, Carson's focus on 143–144
beavers 87–88
bedbugs 104, 105
bees
 Carson aware of 5, 7
 current threat to 4–5, 101–102
 dystopian images 72
 and the gypsy moth Long Island case 92
 in the media 103, 106

Oregon bee-die off (2013) 4, 5
benefits of pesticides
    Carson not entirely opposed to pesticides 70–71, 85, 149, 167
    as line of attack against Carson's work 163–164
Benson, Ezra Taft 164, 166
benzene 135
benzene hexachloride 48, 77
Bhopal explosion (1984) 100
bifenthrin 125
Big Engineering 41–42, 58
Big Pharma 63
Big Science 58
"big picture," need for 26, 35–36
Bihar poisoning 5–6
Bikini atoll experiments 43, 47, 75
bioaccumulation 75–77, 79, 80, 117–118, 120, 131
"biocides" 55, 71
biographical details about Carson 11–18
biological control 33, 147–149, 161
biological resistance 55, 101
biomagnification 74, 75–77, 82, 93
biomonitoring 132
birds
    bird counts 151
    bird deaths 92–96
    as central theme of *Silent Spring* 95
    and chlordane/heptachlor 80
    current situation 99, 104–105
    and DDT spraying 69–70, 137
    as direct targets of pesticides 93
    endocrine disruption 137
    and endrin 82
    hunting using pesticides 103
    as illustration of interconnectedness of nature 86
    no need for direct exposure 75, 77
    pesticides in wild bird food products 104
    in Sheldon, Illinois 89
    and the war against nature 56
black market pesticides 106
"body burden" 127, 131–132
Boehner, John 169
bones
    bone marrow destruction from pesticides 48, 135
    pesticides and radiation ending up in 50, 51
"Boston marriage" 16
botany 18–19
"boys and their toys" 56
brain development 106
brand names 57–58, 114
breast cancer
    Carson's own 2, 11, 109–110
    chlordane linked to 80
    the current breast cancer movement 136–137
    and estrogenic chemicals 136–137
    not mentioned in *Silent Spring* 136
Breast Cancer Action 136
Briggs, Shirley 14
brink, world at the 118–119, 171
Brook, F. 90
Brooks, Paul 10, 25, 159
butter 121
butterflies 105
"bystander" insects 101, 147

calcium absorption 77
Canada
    Minamata disease 62
    Miramichi region spraying 96–98
    and thalidomide 63
cancer *see also* breast cancer
    2,4D as carcinogen 115
    carcinogenicity possibly enhanced by detergents 130

INDEX

in employees at nuclear facilities 119
EPA assessments of carcinogenicity 80, 106, 124
indirect carcinogenesis 137–138
long-term carcinogenic effects unknown 100
"possible carcinogen" status of DDT 168
President's Cancer Panel report 3
in *Silent Spring* 134–138
and the slow wheels of regulation 126
capitalism 23, 28, 32, 41, 84, 164
carbofuran 103
carcinogenic effects of chemicals *see* cancer
cascading/spiraling effects of chemical use 55, 74, 87, 100–101
catalysts for *Silent Spring*
aerial spraying programs 69–70
bird die-off 95
Long Island pesticide misuse case 91–92
cattle farming 87
cause and effect, difficulties in establishing 127, 131, 133, 156

CDC (Centers for Disease Control) 132
"ceilings" and "floors," debate over 132
celery 105
cell damage 52, 131
cellular mutation 138–140
Chemical and Engineering News 164, 165, 166
chemical companies *see* industry (chemical)
chemical fog, humans live in 117, 120, 130–131

chemical transformation 51, 82
chemical weapons 5–6, 53–54
childhood cancers 134
China
continued used of DDT 166
Hebei province chemical explosion 106
suicide by pesticide 6
Chisso Corporation 60–62
chlordane 78–80
banned by EPA 162
half-life 77
as home pesticide 113
toxicity 132
chlorinated hydrocarbons *see also* specific chemicals e.g. DDT
deaths caused by 95
hormonal effects 137–138
in human food 121
and the placenta barrier 74
replacing with naturally-derived ones 147
sensitivity of fish 97
in *Silent Spring* 72, 81
time lag to notice effects 135
chloropyrifos 106
cholera 72
Chomsky, Noam 31
chromosome damage 115, 138–140
chronic effects 99, 119, 120, 133
see also low-level effects of pesticides
"circumstantial," evidence dismissed as 135
citizen science 36, 150–152
civilization and the war metaphor 56
"classic" status of *Silent Spring* 2–3
Clear Lake grebe population 75–77
climate change denials 152–153, 168
CNN 102–106
Coburn, Tom 169–170

INDEX

Colborn, Theo 137
Cold War
   and American culture 43, 53, 68, 70
   Carson critical of 47
   influence on pesticide development 38, 41, 68
collusion, science-industry-government 31–40, 154
colony collapse disorder (CCD) 101, 106
combinations of chemicals *see* synergistic effects of chemicals
Commoner, Barry 46, 154–155
communism
   Carson accused of 32, 164
   Silent Spring linked with communist books 7
compensation for contamination 61
Competitive Enterprise Institute 169
compilation of information, Carson's skills in 68–69
conflicts of interest 35, 37, 60, 65
confusion, public, deliberately created 153
Congressional committee testimony (1963) 115–116, 130, 161
conservative movement 7, 167–168
contacts, Carson's 70
contemporary situation
   biomonitoring studies about current "body burden" 132
   childhood cancers 134
   DDT 166–167, 169–170
   domestic pesticides 116
   food residues 125–126
   food safety regulation 123–124
   lack of knowledge about synergistic effects continues 130
   marketing of home pesticides 112
   pesticide residues in food 59–60, 104–105, 121, 122, 125–126
   precautionary principle 155–157
   Silent Spring still influential 3, 159–172
control of nature ideology
   and the arrogance of "man" 53
   Carson focussed on interconnectedness of humans and nature 127, 145, 148, 152, 172
   contributing to "world at the brink" 118
   and control of women 28–31
   echoed in brand names of pesticides 57–58
   exaggeration of the need for control 39
   masculinized control of nature 57
   as meta-narrative in *Silent Spring* 25–26, 67
   as only recent possibility 50–51
   pesticides both product of and advancing the goals of 68
   and "productionist" values 84
   and science 26–31, 67
   as "stone-age" approach to human-nature relationship 25–26
   war on nature 55–56, 67–68, 73, 148
controversial issues
   2,4-D 115
   Carson's work on chemical mutagenesis 140
   DDT and "floors" and "ceilings" of exposure debate 132

"deadliest sin to be controversial" in 1950s 41
low-level effects of pesticides 119
pesticide residues in food 59–60, 104–105, 121, 122, 125–126
presence and significance of chemical residues in food 121
Silent Spring still highly controversial 7–8, 166–170
Silent Spring written with polemical agenda 144
willful ignorance in government/industry 154
Conway, E. 153–154
core arguments of *Silent Spring* 71–72
Cottam, Clarence 60, 69
Cousteau, Jacques 10–11
crabgrass 114
cranberry crisis 59–60
credibility, Carson's 110 *see also* scientist, Carson as
crowdsourcing 152
cultural outsider, Carson as 25
cumulative effect
  accumulating sequence of poisoning 51, 52, 74, 75–77, 131
  bioaccumulation 75–77, 79, 80, 117–118, 120, 131
  Carson at the cutting edge of science about 127, 131–133
  and the "chemical fog" 120
  of chlorinated hydrocarbons 79
curiosity, Carson bemoans lack of 90, 91
cutting edge, Carson at the
  cancer-environment link 3
  citizen science 150–152
  cumulative effects 127, 131–133

endocrine disruption 137
evidence basis of Carson's work 109, 121
genetics and cellular mutagenesis 138–140
natural controls 147–149
precautionary principle 155–157
synergistic effects of chemicals 126, 127–131, 135–136

Darby, William 165, 166
DDD (DDT compound) and grebe deaths 75–77
DDT
  banning of 162, 166–167, 168
  and bees 5
  and biomagnification 131
  in breastmilk 68
  compared to aldrin/dieldrin/endrin 81, 82, 89
  compared to chlordane/heptachlor 79
  and the conservative movement 167–168
  contemporary situation 78, 125, 167–168
  endocrine disruption in birds 137
  found in everyone's bodies 120–121
  gypsy moth Long Island case 38–39, 56, 70, 91–92, 150–151
  as home pesticide 112–113
  in human food 121, 125
  and the military 54
  Miramichi region spraying 96–98
  for mosquito control 69–70, 168–170
  New York Times joke obituary 166
  as product of wartime science 52

INDEX

renewed calls for use of 169–170
and "safe" doses 135–136
in *Silent Spring* 72–78
Swedish farmer story 48
and the war against nature 56
deaths (human) from chemical exposure
   indirect deaths. *see* bioaccumulation; cancer; food, human; health, human; low-level effects of pesticides
   suicide by pesticide swallowing 6, 7, 103
   threat to those working directly with chemicals 79, 81, 99, 103, 105, 132–133
deception, outright 118
deformities, birth
   in Minamata 61, 62
   thalidomide 63–66
delayed impact of chemical exposure 119, 125, 127, 131, 133, 135
Democrat, Carson as 32
dengue fever 73, 103
Department of Agriculture Yearbook 67, 73
depression 133–134
detergents 130, 136, 137
Detroit, aldrin spraying 94
developing countries 80, 166–170
Dharmasati Gandaman poisoning 5
diazinon 99
dieldrin
   banned by EPA 162
   fire ant eradication programs 69
   in the home 113
   in the human body 132
   salt marsh spraying, Florida 97
   in Sheldon, Illinois 88–89
   in *Silent Spring* 72, 81–83
   still circulating in food system 125
"die-offs"
   bees 4, 101
   birds 75–77, 104–105
   still common 99
dinotefuran 4
dioxins
   EPA dioxin study 106, 124
   Seveso disaster 100
"Dirty Dozen" list 125
diseases
   Carson on insect-borne disease 167
   disease outcomes from chemical exposure 133–140 *see also* cancer
   pesticides used to prevent 54
   using natural disease to control insects 147
Disney wallpaper 112
distanced effect of chemical exposure 127, 131, 133
distribution mechanisms
   air currents transport 82
   Carson particularly against aerial spraying 69–71, 89–92
   marine systems 48–9, 97
   of endocrine disruptors 137
   of radioactive poisoning in marine ecosystems 48–49
   unpredictability of wind/water transfer 51
   via birds 93
   water systems 54
Dole 105
dolphins 105
domestic markets
   DDT moving from military to domestic markets 73
   household pesticides 98, 104, 105, 111–113
doubt, as industrial strategy 153
Dow 99, 106
Drew, E. 42, 43

drugs
    drug companies 63
    regulation of drugs higher than pesticides 115
    unknown combined effects of drugs and pesticides 130
Dryden Chemicals 62
dual dominance (men over women and nature) ideology 29
DuPont 10, 99
Dutch elm disease 151
duties of ordinary citizens 34–35, 150–152
dystopia 72, 118, 171

eagles 77
Earthwatch expeditions 151
easy life pursuit of threatens entire planet 30
ecology
    Army Corps of Engineers on 42
    Carson introduces concept of "ecology of the body" 127
    Carson's readers familiar with 86
    dominant role of science in the ecological crisis 27
Ecology of Invasions of Animals and Plants, The (Elton, 1958) 84
economics *see also* profit, pursuit of
    economic damage caused by collateral spraying 97
    strong economy and the need for pesticides 98
ecosystems
    Carson introduces concept to readers 83–89
    Carson's ecosystem analysis of aquatic environments 96–98
    ecosystem poisoning in atomic age 48–49, 75

Edge of the Sea (Carson, 1955) 10, 13
education, Carson's goal of 34–35, 36, 83, 138, 150–152
effects of *Silent Spring*
    banning of DDT 162, 166–167, 168
    banning of organochlorine pesticides 92
    as baseline for today's environmental movement 159
    the breast cancer movement 136
    Carson did not live to see 2
    Carson offers hope 143–146
    Carson's concerns are still with us 99
    citizen science 150–152
    in the current bee issue 4
    development of "integrated pest management" 148
    early warnings about endocrine disruption 138
    further research into effect on raptors 77
    idea of ecology of the body 127
    link between health and environment 111
    public awareness 161
    public health concerns about chemicals in food 121
    regulation of chemicals revised 161–162
    Silent Spring as a "classic" 2–3
    synergistic effects of chemicals 130–131
    vindication by President's Science Advisory Committee 161
Einstein, Albert 46
Eiseley, Loren 40
Eisenhower, Dwight 33–34, 36, 46, 54, 164
Elton, Charles 83, 84, 91

endocrine disruption 137–138
endrin 81–83, 162
engineering
  Big Engineering 56–57
  masculine nature of 56–57
  post-war engineering projects 41–42
Enloe, Cynthia 57
entomology 25, 33
environmental movement 20, 28, 136
Environmental Working Group 125
EPA (Environmental Protection Agency)
  acknowledgement of synergistic effects 127–128
  and aldrin/dieldrin/endrin 82–83
  approved chemicals (current) 98
  and chlordane/heptachlor 79, 80
  and DDT 166–167
  dioxin study 106, 124
  establishment in 1970 161–162
  and GMO crops 101
  inadequacy of 116, 124
  and IPM 148
estrogenic chemicals 82, 136–138
EU (European Union)
  on GM crops 101
  on neonicotinoids 4, 102
  and the precautionary principle 157
European Renaissance science 26–27
evidence bases
  about food 121
  on cancer 134
  Carson at the frontier of medical evidence 109, 121
  Carson believes facts do exist 35
  Carson did not conduct original research 68
  Carson highlights gaps 81
  Carson's evidence attacked post-publication 163
  continued use of pesticides despite lack of information 116, 123, 126, 152
  evidence basis for pesticides still lacking now 116–117
  evidence dismissed as "circumstantial" 135
  and persistence of chemicals 77–78
  pointing towards cause and effect of pesticide poisoning 133–140
  "translation" of scientific literature by Carson 68, 83, 109, 131–132
evil, Carson on 51, 52, 87
excretion of pesticides from the body 74, 132
experiments on people 126, 130–131, 152

fable, town 24, 50, 87, 145–146, 163–164
Faderman, Lillian 16, 17
false assurances to public 32, 35, 118, 154
false claims 116–117
Farm Chemicals magazine 165–166
fast-tracking chemicals to market 123
fat solubility 75, 120, 121, 137
fatty foodstuffs as greatest concentrators of pesticides 75
fatty tissue storage 74, 76, 80, 81, 120, 128
FDA (Food and Drug Administration)
  malathion study 128
  and pesticide residues in food 59–60, 121, 122, 125–126
  and thalidomide 63–64, 65

Federal Insecticide, Fungicide, and Rodenticide Act (FIFRA) 162
Federal Radiation Council 46
Feminine Mystique (Friedan, 1963) 7, 30, 114
femininity *see also* gender; women
   earth as nurturing mother 27
   Kelsey as "feminine" conscience of FDA 65
   nature as female 29
   study of nature socially acceptable for women 18–19
feminism 13, 17–20, 26–31
   devaluation of women compared to devaluation of nature 28–29
   and the environmental causes of breast cancer 136
   feminist environmental analysis 29
   feminist technology studies 56–57
   no feminist analysis in *Silent Spring* 30, 118–119
   and science 29, 13, 17–20, 26–31
fine print, details of pesticides hidden in 114
fire ant eradication programs 38–39, 69, 79, 91
fish
   and bioaccumulation 76
   and DDT/heptachlor 79
   economic damage to fishing industry 97
   Florida salt marsh spraying 97
   Miramichi region spraying 96–98
Fish and Wildlife Service 12–13, 60, 68, 69, 111
"flareback" 74, 89
"floors" and "ceilings," debate over 132
Florida salt marsh spraying 97

fludioxonil 125
food, human
   cranberry contamination crisis 59–60
   food allergies 103
   food safety regulation 59–60, 121, 122–123
   humans at top of bioaccumulating food chain 120
   pesticide residues in food 59–60, 104–105, 121, 122, 125–126
   school lunch poisoning, India 5
   as source of chemical poisoning 121–126
   surplus food 84
food chains and bioaccumulation 75–77, 86, 89, 117–118, 120
foresight, need for 154–155
Freeman, Dorothy 11, 14–16
Friedan, Betty 7, 30, 114
frontiers of science, Carson at
   cancer-environment link 3
   citizen science 150–152
   cumulative effects 127, 131–133
   endocrine disruption 137
   evidence basis of Carson's work 109, 121
   genetics and cellular mutagenesis 138–140
   natural controls 147–149
   precautionary principle 155–157
   synergistic effects of chemicals 126, 127–131, 135–136
Fundamentals of Ecology (Odum, 1953) 11
funding
   into the "body burden" 132
   Carson becoming suspicious about 60
   influence of funding on entomology 33

INDEX

lack of funding for research into effects 90, 154
more money available for pesticide research than biological 33
science-industry-government collusion 31–40

GAO (US Government Accountability Office) 116, 124
gardening, pesticides for 112, 113–114 *see also* household pesticides
gateway drug, DDT as 72–74
gender *see also* masculine hegemonies; misogyny; sexism
    gender analysis nascent in Carson's work although not explicit 30, 56–57
    gender identity manipulation and home pesticide marketing 111–114
    gendered views of areas of scientific study 18–19
    triumph of male science over female nature 29, 165
    used to attack Carson 164–166
generational transmission 74, 76–77, 138
genetic mutations 52, 53, 65–66
genetics 138–140
glyphosate 125
GMOs (genetically modified crops) 100–101, 106
governments
    Carson as "translator" of government information 68
    Carson exposes lack of government protection re food 122
    on domestication of pesticides 113
    government secrecy 45, 47

government-industry collusion 32–33, 123, 126
Japanese government in Minamata disease 61
science-industry-government collusion 31–40
shirking duty as neutral arbiters of truth 35
uncurious about wide-ranging effects of pesticides 90
US government in cranberry crisis 59–60
US government response to *Silent Spring* 160–161
and willful ignorance 154
grebes dying off 75–77
greed *see* profit, pursuit of
"green run" experiment 44
Grunwald, M. 42
guinea pig, public as 126, 130–131, 152
gypsy moths
    pheromone manipulation 147
    spraying programs (Long Island) 38–39, 56, 70, 91–92, 150–151

habit of killing 3, 54, 55, 71, 90
half truths 85
half-life statistics 77
Hanford reservation (atomic city) 44, 119
Haraway, Donna 29
Harding, Sandra 19, 29
hazard warnings (on packaging) 55, 113
Hazlett, M. 18, 165, 166
health, human
    Carson made link between health and ecologies 110–111, 126–133 *see also* cancer; diseases; food, human; low-level effects of pesticides
    Carson's own health 109

health-based tolerance levels for food (lack of) 123
Hebei province chemical explosion 106
heptachlor 69, 79–80, 162
Herber, Lewis 11
herbicides *see* pesticides
heredity *see* genetics
Hiroshima attack 43
Hitchcock, Alfred 1–2
"holocaust," Carson's (single) use of the word 96–97
honor killings by pesticide 6
hope, Carson offers 143–146
Horkheimer, Max 28
hormonal system, disruption to 137
Houghton Mifflin 10
household pesticides 98, 104, 105, 111–112
household products as endocrine disruptors 137
Huckins, Olga Owens 14, 70, 95, 150
humility, loss of 144–145
hunting, pesticides for 103
Hynes, Patricia 20, 31, 53, 69

ignorance, willful 118, 154
imagination, lack of 118
inattention (of citizens) 34–35, 118
India
　Bhopal explosion (1984) 100
　Bihar poisoning 5
　continued used of DDT 166
　"drowning in pesticides" 6, 7
indirect exposure rarer than direct 119
indiscriminate use of pesticides
　automaticity of use of insecticides 89–90
　Carson particularly against 69–71, 87, 89–92
　and damage to aquatic environments 97
　direct effect on people 92
　direct effect on wildlife 89, 92
　vs IPM 148–149
　vs natural controls 147, 148
　and "pesticide drift" 89, 90–92, 103
　pesticides as routine 30
industrial accidents 99–100, 106
industrial workers, threats to 119, 132, 133
industrialization 23
industry (chemical)
　attacks on Carson 163
　continued animosity towards Carson 167
　current situation 99
　industry-created scientific uncertainty 152–157
　industry-government collusion 32–33, 123, 126
　influencing entomological research with funding 33
　pollution local to factories 53–54
　radical realignment of priorities in the precautionary principle 156
　science-industry-government collusion 31–40
influences on Carson 14
　Charles Elton 84
　Clarence Cottam 60, 69
　Dorothy Freeman 11, 14–16
　Marie Rodell 14, 20–21
　Marjorie Spock 14, 70, 92
　Mary (Polly) Richards 70, 92
　Mary Scott Skinker 12, 14
　Olga Owens Huckins 14, 70, 95
　Robert Rudd 84
information and knowledge
　Carson as "translator" of government information 68
　Carson as "translator" of scientific literature 68, 83, 109, 131–132

Carson refers frequently to lack of 152
continued use of pesticides despite lack of information 81, 82, 116, 123, 126, 152
making decisions on incomplete information 110
public policy waits for surety before acting 152–153
scientific uncertainty 152–157
well known nervous system effects 133
willful ignorance 118, 154
informed citizens
as best defence against military-industrial complex 34
Carson caters for lay readers 83, 131, 137, 138, 150–152
citizen science 36, 150–152
classified information 45
duties of ordinary citizens 34–35, 150–152
pulled between competing accounts 35–36
innovations in Carson's work
advocacy of natural controls 148
calls for genetic testing 65–66
citizen science 36, 150–152
concept of "ecology of the body" 127
ecosystems 83–89
focus on low-level effects of pesticides 3, 119–126
genetics 138–139
military-pesticide link 7
mutagenesis of chemicals/genetics 138–140
inorganic mercury 60–62
insecticides *see* pesticides
institutional relationships
and the crisis of confidence 65
Kelsey's efforts to buck system 63

science-industry-government collusion 37
interactions, chemical 127–131
interconnectedness
aquatic environments 96–98
Carson's ecosystem thinking 85–86, 87
human health and the environment 110, 127
humans-nature 85, 127, 145, 148, 172
and loss of humility in modern life 144
novelty of idea in 1960s 54
Internet and citizen science 152
interviews with Carson on CBS 26
intimate relationship between Carson and Freeman 11, 14–16
iodine, radioactive 44
IPM (integrated pest management) 148
irreversibility of environmental damage 51
Ishimure, Michiko 62
Italy, Seveso disaster 100

Japan
and DDT spraying 73
"Lucky Dragon" catastrophe 47–48
Minamata disease 60–62
Japanese beetle 88–89, 90, 94, 147

Keller, Evelyn Fox 18, 29
Kelsey, Dr Frances 63–64
Kemm, K. 168–169
Kennedy, John F. 160
kidney damage 74, 104
killing, habit of 3, 54, 55, 71, 90
kitchen shelf paper 112–113
Klamath weed 147
knowledge *see* informaiton and knowledge

INDEX

language used by Carson
   "biocides" 55, 71
   "carnage" 97
   "ecology of the body" 127
   "ecosystem" 83–89
   habit of killing 3, 54, 55, 71, 90
   "holocaust" 96–97
   "humility" 144–145
   "misfortune" 145–146
   no brand names 57–58
   not generally alarmist 140
   phrases indicating "uncertainty" 152
last resort, pesticides should be 148
lawn care 99, 111–112, 114, 115
lay readers, Carson caters for 83, 131, 137, 138, 150–152
LD-50 testing 122
Lear, Linda 12, 14, 15, 19, 20, 25, 40, 52, 69, 92, 109, 159–160
left-leaning thinkers, Carson amongst 32, 84, 168
legal action
   against aerial spraying (Long Island) 92, 150–151
   post-*Silent Spring* 78–79, 162
   threatened pre-*Silent Spring* 10
Lehman, Dr 79
"lesbian" relationship, Carson and Freeman 15–16
letters, Carson's
   to Catherine Scott 20
   to Clarence Cottam re cranberry crisis 60
   to Dorothy Freeman 15–16
   to *New York Times* 1959 84
letters to the editor
   about Carson 164
   and aerial spraying programs 151
leukemia 134–135, 136
liability
   denied by drug companies for thalidomide 63

Japanese government in Minamata disease 61–62
lice 73
life, threat to all
   all forms of life under threat 52, 55
   lack of regard for life 90
   threat to human life generally from chemicals 49, 52, 98, 99
lindane 113, 133, 135
livelihoods, damage to 97
liver damage 74, 81, 135, 138
Long Island pesticide misuse case 38–39, 56, 70, 91–92, 150–151
longitudinal studies 132
long-term impacts, lack of research into 81
looking the other way 34–35
low-level effects of pesticides
   Carson focuses on 3, 119–126
   delayed impact of chemical exposure 119, 125, 127, 131, 133, 135
   distanced effect of chemical exposure 127, 131, 133
   lack of understanding about far-reaching effects of contamination 49, 81
   as marginal area of research 120
"Lucky Dragon" catastrophe 47–48
Lysenkoism 38

Machine in the Garden, The (Marx, 1956) 23–24
machines
   Leo Marx on 23–24
   as metaphor for nature 27
   militaries, militarism, and the atomic world 40–58
   Silent Spring as manifesto against 24

INDEX

malaria
    and DDT 54, 69–70, 73, 78, 166–167
    and dieldrin 81
    resurgence blamed on Carson 168, 170
malathion 128–129
man against nature *see* control of nature ideology
"manufacturing consent" 31
marginalization, of Carson's work 120 *see also* frontiers of science, Carson at
marine ecosystems
    mercury contamination 61
    radioactive poisoning of 48–49
    in *Silent Spring* 96–98
marketing
    effects of 35
    of home pesticides 111–117
    of *Silent Spring* 160
Marx, Karl 32
Marx, Leo 23–24
masculine hegemonies
    "boys and their toys" 56
    the capitalist norm vs Carson's "caring" 164
    dual dominance (men over women and nature) ideology 29
    military and engineering 56–57
    nuclear power and pesticide power derive from "man's" arrogance 53
    and risk-taking 118–119
    of science 29 *see also* Baconian science
    women-home vs men-outdoors in pesticide marketing 111–112, 113–114
mass experimentation, pesticide use as 126, 130–131, 152
mass-production 54, 74
media coverage
    1950s warnings about global warming 11
    2012, pesticide news in 102–103
    cranberry crisis (1959) 59–60
    of the crisis of confidence in institutions 65
    of Minamata disease 62
    of *Silent Spring* 160
    Silent Spring still mentioned today 5
Melbourne study (mental illness) 133
memory loss 133–134
mental illness 133
Merchant, Carolyn 27, 28–29, 30, 32
Merchants of Doubt (Oreskes and Conway, 2010) 153
mercury contamination 60–62
Merrell 63–64
meta-narratives of *Silent Spring* 24, 25–26, 152
metaphors
    chemical fog 117, 120, 130–131
    mechanistic metaphors for nature 27
    "rain of death" 84, 88, 89–92
    war against nature 55–56, 67–68, 73, 148
Metcalf, Robert 165
methyl iodide 103, 106
methylmercury 60–62
middle classes
    and citizen science 151
    and home pesticide use 112–114
military, the
    allure of militarized power 118
    Carson not directly critical of 54
    chemical weapons 5–6, 53–54
    and control of nature 41–43
    DDT as military weapon 73
    masculine nature of 56–57
    militarism 54

militarism and the war on nature 55–58, 67–68, 73, 148
militarized view of human-nature relationship 7, 54–56
military technology 40–58
military-industrial complex 33–34, 37, 54
military-pesticide link 7, 40–58
in post-WWII America 43, 53, 58, 68, 70
milk
  irradiated 46, 47
  pesticide residues banned in 121
  pesticides in breastmilk 68, 118
milky spore disease 147
Minamata disease 60–62
Miracle-Gro 104
Miramichi region spraying 96–98
"misfortune" 145–146
misogyny see also sexism
  against Carson 11, 13, 17, 164–166
  male doctor-woman patient 109–110
  against Stewart 119
  women as "other" 29
  against women in science 17–20, 26–31
  women-home vs men-outdoors in pesticide marketing 111–112, 113–114
modernism 29, 35
modernity
  Carson notes high price of 30
  pesticide use as sign of 112–114
monocrotophos 5
Monsanto 99, 100–101, 163
moose 87–88
morality
  Carson questions humanity's 50

"family values" and the use of domestic pesticides 112–113
human values 84–85, 163
humanity diminished by acquiescence to causing suffering 95
moral bankruptcy of food safety regulation 122–123
mosquitos
  and DDT (as prevention) 69, 73, 167, 169–170
  and dieldrin 81
  home pesticides for 105, 113
moth killers 113
mother earth 27
mothering, pesticides marketed as part of "good" 112
Muller, Hermann 138, 139, 140
multiple chemical exposure 128
  see also synergistic effects of chemicals
murder by pesticide (honor killings) 6
Murphy, Robert Cushman 70
mutagenic effects 138–140
mutations, chemical 51, 82

narratives
  Carson uses stories to make her points 83, 86–89
  meta-narratives of Silent Spring 24, 25–26, 152
  reliability of narrators 35
  science and false narratives 30
  Western "mastery" of nature narrative 30
National Academy of Science/National Research Council 69
natural controls 147–149, 161
Natural Resources Defense Council 80
nature
  Baconian scientific views of 28
  in a capitalist system 32

INDEX

Carson as a nature-writer 9, 10, 17–18, 144
Carson's love of as source for criticism 164, 165
control of nature *see* control of nature ideology
ecosystems 83–89
as female 29
and industrialization/the "machine" 23
interconnectedness of humans and nature 85, 127, 145, 148, 172
moves more slowly than fast pace of new chemicals 51
"nature awareness" and citizen science 150–152
pivotal shift of scientific views of in sixteenth and seventeenth centuries 27, 30
study of nature socially acceptable for women 18
war against nature 55–56, 67–68, 73, 148
wonder, beauty, and passion 143–146
need
approval for use should be needs-based 39
growth in pesticide use not based on 111
manufactured "need" for pesticides 39
neonicotinoids 4, 102, 106
nerve gases 53, 54
nervous system disorders 133–134
neurological damage
from 2,4D 115–116
brain development 106
from mercury (in Minamata) 60
New York Times
2012 coverage of pesticides 102–106

Carson's letters to 84
Carson's obituary 17
coverage of cranberry crisis 59
coverage of Kelsey 65
joke obituary of DDT 166
on *Silent Spring* 40
New Yorker
letters about Carson 164
serialization of *Silent Spring* 9–10, 159, 160, 162
Niigata, Japan 61
Noble, D. 29
non-Hodgkin's lymphoma 115
Norfolk, England 94
nothing, doing (as alternative) 156
novelty, pursuit of 56, 118
nuclear power 43–58, 119
"nun of nature," Carson referred to as 17

O'Brien, W. 42
obstructionism 64
oceans *see* marine ecosystems
Odum, Eugene 11, 83
oil companies 53
optimism, Carson's 143
Oreskes, N. 153–154
organic food debate 104
organic pest control 33, 147–149, 161
organophosphates
Carson on accidental contact with 7
and chemical weapons 5–6
and long-term damage 133
now considered "old" pesticides 5
organic phosphorus pesticides 72, 99
and suicides 6
and synergistic effects 128–129
"other road," the 146, 155
Our Stolen Future (Colbourn, 1996) 137

INDEX

Our Synthetic Environment (Herber, 1962) 11
over-emotional, Carson accused of being 165
overnight sensation, *Silent Spring* as 66
overproduction 84
Oxford University Press 20

paint, pesticides in 105
paralysis 133
parathion 7, 72, 93
passivity, not found in *Silent Spring* 30–31
pastoral ideals 23–24
patriarchies *see* masculine hegemonies
Pearson, Drew 60
permanency of environmental damage 51
persistence of chemicals 77–78, 82, 83, 120, 131
Peru dolphin deaths 105
pessimism, concerns dismissed as 56
pesticide drift 89, 90–92, 103
pesticides *see also* aerial spraying programs; indiscriminate use of pesticides; *specific chemicals*
   brand names 57–58
   Carson not entirely opposed to 70–71, 85, 149, 167
   Carson's history of concern over 69–70
   contemporary situation 78, 79–80, 82–83, 98–106
   and the control of nature (meta-narrative) 25
   and GMO crops 100–101
   household pesticides 98, 104, 105, 111–112
   in human food 59–60, 104–105, 121, 122, 125–126
   military origins 54
   more money available for research (than biological) 33
   naturally-derived pesticides 147
   parallel between chemicals and radioactivity 48, 50–54, 75, 134–136, 138, 139, 140
   parallel between pesticides and thalidomide 66
   pesticide producers and wanton disregard for life 90
   as by-product of war 54
pest-resistant varieties 100–101, 106, 149
"pests," definition of 31
pheromone manipulation 147, 149
phocomelia 63
placenta, pesticides travelling through 74, 118
plankton 76
planning, Carson attacks lack of 90
plants
   all life depends on 144
   lawn care 99, 111–112, 114, 115
   natural plant control 147
   plant killing chemicals 144
   selective spraying 149–150
   weed killers 144
Plass, Gilbert 11
plastics 137
Plumwood, Val 29
plutonium 43, 44
Pogo (comic strip character) 2
political affiliation, Carson's
   accused of communism 32, 164
   conservative movement response to *Silent Spring* 7, 167–168
   criticized as "un-American" 111, 164
   Democrat 32
   left-leaning thinkers, Carson amongst 32, 84, 168
pollination 101–102

INDEX

POPs (Persistent Organic Pollutants) 78, 80, 82, 166
popularized science, *Silent Spring* as 137
potentiated toxicity 128
precautionary principle 3, 155–157
predictability of results of pesticide use, Carson's outrage over 97
President's Cancer Panel report 3
pressure tactics 64
prevention strategies 149
privacy, Carson's own 109
production
  misplaced prioritization of 84, 122
  overproduction 84
profit, pursuit of
  Carson denouncing 37, 39, 84–85, 163
  and controversial industries 153
  and the move to domestic pesticides 111
  and risk-taking 118
  and the science-industry-government collusion 31–32
  as subtext of *Silent Spring* 39–40
  tension between economy and threat to life 98
"progress"
  Carson challenges 25, 30, 68, 163, 172
  "rational man" argument for progress 42
  as subtext of *Silent Spring* 40
  women as victims of scientific progress 30
proof *see also* evidence bases
  burden of proof should be on proponent not public 156
  Carson could not prove cause and effect 133
proprietary names 57–58, 114

PSAC (President's Science Advisory Committee) 160–161, 163
public health concerns 121
Public Health Service 69
public policy and scientific uncertainty 152–157
publishing, Carson's interest in 20
"Pugwash" meeting 46
pyrethins 147

questioning/curiosity, Carson bemoans lack of 90, 91

Rachel Was Wrong website 169
radicalism in *Silent Spring* 31, 85
radioactivity
  atomic world 44–53
  and bioaccumulation 75–77
  and cellular mutation 138
  combinations of chemicals and radiation 129–130
  concerns over low-level exposure 119
  parallel between chemicals and radioactivity 48, 50–54, 75, 134–136, 138, 139, 140
  from plutonium production 44–45
"rain of death" 84, 88, 89–92
raptors (top of the food chain) 77
rationalist worldviews 28, 29, 42, 165
readership, Carson's dual 9, 83, 85
"rebounds" 71, 74, 89
RECA (Radiation Exposure Compensation Act) 45–46
received wisdom, Carson questioned 25, 40
recklessness, humans' 50, 51, 54, 71, 84
redundancy of pesticides 39
regulatory systems *see also* EPA; FDA
  for aerial spraying 92

on behalf of birds 99
corruption of regulatory-industry relationship 118
do not cover genetic effect 140
for food 121, 122–124, 125–126
for GMO crops 101
of home pesticides 114–115
inadequacy of 71
influenced by *Silent Spring* 3, 161–162
for neonicotinoids 102
and scientific uncertainty 152–153
Reiss, Louise and Eric 46
relationships, Carson's personal *see also* influences on Carson
dependent family 11, 14
female friends 14
with her mother 12, 16
intimate relationship with Dorothy Freeman 11, 14–16
remaining unmarried ("spinsterhood") 16–18
"reliable narrator," Carson's search for 35
religion, lack of in *Silent Spring* 145
Renaissance science 26–27
reproductive systems 77, 82, 100, 115, 137
research *see* evidence bases
research institutes, and the influence of chemical companies 33
resistance, biological 55, 71, 72, 74, 167
reviews of *Silent Spring* 2, 40, 159–166
Ribicoff hearings 161
Richards, Mary 70, 92
rights 31, 35
right-wing movements 7, 167–168
risk assessment 154, 155
risk-taking 118–119

rivers, control of 42
road less traveled/the "other road" 146, 155
Robson, William 139
Rocky Mountain Arsenal pollution scandal 53–54
Rodell, Marie 14, 20–21, 159–160
Rorschach test, *Silent Spring* as 7
rotenone 147
Roundup-ready soybeans 100–101
Rudd, Robert 84–85
runoff, threat from 97, 100
Russell, Bertrand 46
Russia 43, 44

"Safari" 4
sagebrush eradication program 86–88
salad 128–129
salt marsh spraying, Florida 97
sampling (food safety) 122–123, 124, 125
Sandoz chemical spill (1986) 100
sarin 5–6
school lunch poisoning, India 5
Schrader, Gerhard 54
Schweitzer, Albert 51
science *see also* frontiers of science, Carson at
Carson not anti-science 144, 165
Carson on "democratized" science 36
Carson writes for the scientific establishment 83
citizen science 150–152
and the "control of nature" ideology 26–31, 67
damage done by extreme specialization 35–36
dominant role of science in ecological crisis 27
and "expert" doubters 153
and false narratives 30
"gender and genre" 19

"good" vs "bad" science 165, 168
history of science 26–31
industry attacks on the science in Carson's work 163
insensate logic of 118
masculinization 26–31
presumption of scientific objectivity 33
and the production of new "weapons" 25–26
and rationality 165
science-industry-government collusion 31–40
scientific "thrill" of pesticide production 111
scientific uncertainty 152–157
as "superior" to nature 27
and the suppression of wonder 143–144
"translation" of scientific literature by Carson 68, 83, 109, 131–132
unable to cope with multiple combinations of chemicals 131
women in 12, 13, 17–20, 26–31
Science for the People 151
Science in Farming (DA Yearbook 1943–1947) 67, 73
"Scientific Revolution" 27, 30
scientist, Carson as
  also able to appreciate beauty and wonder 144
  attacked post-publication 163, 164
  on cancers 134
  on cellular mutation 138
  and the cranberry scare 60
  focused on cumulative effects 131–132
  focused on low-level impacts 120–121
  and gender barriers 19
  and her own ill health 109
  no original research 68 *see also* "translation" of scientific literature
  rarity of women in senior science positions 13
  seen by critics as incompatible with love of nature 164
  Silent Spring as culmination of many years of work 69
  writing for dual readership 9, 83
Scott, Catherine 20
Scott's 104
screw-worm fly 147
Sea Around Us, The (Carson, 1961) 10, 13, 17, 20, 49, 75, 154
Seager, Joni 29, 42, 136
seas *see* marine ecosystems
seeds, treating with insecticides 94
seizures and convulsions 81, 95
selective spraying 149–150
Sense of Wonder, The (Carson, 1965) 145
Seveso disaster (1976) 100
sexism *see also* misogyny
  against Carson 11, 13, 16–20, 17, 29, 164–166
  male doctor-woman patient 109–110
  against Stewart 111–112, 113–114, 119
  against women in science 17–20, 26–31
Shawn, William 10
Sheldon, Illinois poisoning 88–89, 90, 95
Shell Chemical Company 4, 53
Shepard, Paul 118
Shiva, Vandana 6, 29
shock factor in Carson's work
  food as source of chemical poisoning 121–126
  graphic descriptions of wildlife dying 93–94

on persistence of chemicals in environment 77
shout lines 25
Shteir, Ann 18, 19
silence
   Carson's re: her own health 109
   silence of the birds as central trope of *Silent Spring* 95
   silent mechanisms of pesticides and radiation 50
   in the title of the book 1–2
"Silent Spring Institute" 136
Silent World, The (Cousteau, 1953) 10–11
skin absorption 81
Skinker, Mary Scott 12, 14
skull and crossbones marking 55
Smith, Eugene and Aileen 62
soil-based environments
   accumulating sequence of poisoning 77–78
   shorter half-lives than water 77
Soviet science 38
soybeans 100–101, 125
specificity in *Silent Spring* 30–31
speeches, Carson's
   citing of Barry Commoner's work 154–155
   citing of Kelsey's work 65–66
   Garden Club of America 1963 71–72
   to *Herald Tribune* Luncheon 19
   Kaiser Foundation Hospitals (1963) 48–49
   Women's National Press Club (1962) 37–38
speed of development, Carson concerned over 71
spinster, Carson stereotyped as 11, 14, 16–18, 166
spiraling/cascading effects of chemical use 55, 74, 87, 100–101
Spock, Marjorie 14, 70, 92

spraying programs *see* aerial spraying programs
Springdale post office naming 169
Sprow, Ida 14
"St. Louis Committee for Nuclear Information" 46, 50
standpoint theory 19
status quo, supporting the 152
Stein, Gertrude 12
Steingraber, Sandra 2–3, 130–131
sterility
   as goal 31, 118
   sterilized insect populations 147
Stewart, Alice 119
Stockholm Convention on Persistent Organic Pollutants 78, 80, 82, 83, 166, 170
Stoll, M. 164
stories, Carson using to make her points 83, 86–89
stress, and activation of stored pesticides 81
strontium-90 47, 50, 51, 134
suburbia, toxicities of 114
sugar coating of facts 32
suicide by pesticide swallowing 6, 7, 103
Sumimoto Chemicals 4
sunlight, chemicals broken down by 82, 83
"Superfund site" 53–54
Surpassing the Love of Men (Faderman, 1981) 16
surplus food 84
Swainson's hawks 99
Swedish farmer story 48
Switzerland, Sandoz chemical spill 100
synergistic effects of chemicals 126, 127–131, 135–136
Syngenta 99
Syria 5–6

systemic threats, vs localized 48–49

Tansley, Arthur 83
termite control 79, 82
testing
   of chemicals *see* evidence bases
   of drugs 64
   nuclear 43, 47–48
thalidomide 63–66
thresholds
   "ceilings" and "floors," debate over 132
   in IPM (integrated pest management) 148–149
   tolerances-and-samples system 122–126, 129–130
titles for *Silent Spring*, alternative proposed 25
tolerance levels 135
tolerances-and-samples system 122–126, 129–130
town fable 24, 50, 87, 145–146, 163–164
toxaphene 77, 97
Toxic Substances and Disease Registry 82–83
"translation" of scientific literature 9, 68, 83, 109, 131–132
translations of *Silent Spring* 2, 160
trapping pests 149
"tree-hugger" type criticisms of Carson 164–165
triggers for *Silent Spring*
   aerial spraying programs 69–70
   bird die-off 95
   Long Island pesticide misuse case 91–92
trivial uses for pesticides 114
Trost, Cathy 40–41, 164
truth, screening of 35, 38, 85
2,4-D 72, 115–116, 125, 139
2008 global financial crisis 118–119typhus 54, 72

ubiquitousness of chemicals 117, 128
un-American, Carson's work as 111, 164
unborn children
   pesticides in tissues 118
   potential damage from X-rays 119
uncertainty, consistent theme in *Silent Spring* 152–157
Under the Sea-wind (Carson, 1941) 12
understaffing
   of EPA 116, 124
   of FDA 123
   of government agencies generally 124
university scientists 33, 36–37
unpredictability of effects of pesticides 35, 51, 126, 127–131, 135–136
uranium industry 45
US Fish and Wildlife Service 12–13, 60, 68, 69, 111
US Public Heath Survey 121
USDA (US Department of Agriculture)
   annual reports of food sampling 125
   and the cranberry scare 59
   Department of Agriculture Yearbook 67, 73
   and the EPA 162
   fire ant eradication programs 69
   and food safety regulation 124
   and GMO crops 101
   Home and Garden Bulletins 113
   political fallout from *Silent Spring* 162–163

Valent USA 4
values, human 84–85, 112–113, 163
Velsicol 10, 78–79, 80
vested interests 35, 37, 60

Walker, K. 152, 153
wallpaper, DDT impregnated 112
Walsh, L. 152, 153
war against nature 55–56, 67–68, 73, 148
  and militarism 55–56, 67–68, 73, 148
warnings, product 55, 113
water *see also* marine ecosystems
  2,4-D in 125
  chemicals/radiation distributed by water system 51, 54
  and combinations of chemicals/radiation 129–130
  contamination by radioactive iodine 44
  and food chain bioaccumulation 76
  mercury contamination in Mimimata 61
  pesticides in tap water 103
  pollution from pesticide manufacturing 53–54
  sagebrush spraying and lake 87–88
way of life, defending 30–31, 41
weapons, chemical 5–6, 53–54
weed control
  natural plant control 147
  and selective spraying 149–150
West Nile virus 104
WHO (World Health Organization) 81, 166–167, 170
willful ignorance 118, 154
Wilsonville bees 4
Wingspread Conference on the Precautionary Principle 155
witch, Carson portrayed as 165–166

women *see also* feminism; gender; misogyny
  assumed incompatibility of women and science 29
  Carson's relationships with 14–16
  control by men compared to domination of nature 29
  as primary focus of home pesticide marketing 112–113
  as victims of scientific progress 30
  "Women's Strike for Peace" movement 46–47
  in the workplace in 1950s 13
women in science *see also* science; scientist, Carson as
  Alice Stewart 119
  Dr Frances Kelsey (thalidomide) 63–65
  and the environmental movement 20
  as outsiders in science 17–20, 26–31
  in science professions 13, 18–19
  and Woods Hole laboratory 12
women's health movement 109, 136
"Women's Strike for Peace" movement 46–47
wonder, Carson's focus on 143–144
Woods Hole Marine Biological Laboratory 12
working titles for *Silent Spring* 25

X-rays 119, 136

Year of the Flood, The (Atwood, 2009) 171